A Global Perspective/Health Inequity in Heart Failure

Editors

PABLO F. CASTRO
NAOKI SATO
ROBERT J. MENTZ
OVIDIU CHIONCEL

HEART FAILURE CLINICS

www.heartfailure.theclinics.com

Consulting Editors
MANDEEP R. MEHRA
JAVED BUTLER

Founding Editor
JAGAT NARULA

October 2015 • Volume 11 • Number 4

ELSEVIER

1600 John F. Kennedy Boulevard • Suite 1800 • Philadelphia, Pennsylvania, 19103-2899

http://www.theclinics.com

HEART FAILURE CLINICS Volume 11, Number 4
October 2015 ISSN 1551-7136, ISBN-13: 978-0-323-40086-2

Editor: Lauren Boyle
Developmental Editor: Alison Swety

Heart Failure Clinics (ISSN 1551-7136) is published quarterly by Elsevier Inc., 360 Park Avenue South, New York, NY 10010-1710. Months of publication are January, April, July, and October. Business and editorial offices: 1600 John F. Kennedy Boulevard, Suite 1800, Philadelphia, PA 19103-2899. Periodicals postage paid at New York, NY, and additional mailing offices. Subscription prices are USD 235.00 per year for US individuals, USD 382.00 per year for US institutions, USD 80.00 per year for US students and residents, USD 280.00 per year for Canadian individuals, USD 442.00 per year for Canadian institutions, USD 300.00 per year for international individuals, USD 442.00 per year for international institutions, and USD 100.00 per year for Canadian and foreign students/residents. To receive student and resident rate, orders must be accompanied by name of affiliated institution, date of term, and the *signature* of program/residency coordinator on institution letterhead. Orders will be billed at individual rate until proof of status is received. Foreign air speed delivery is included in all *Clinics* subscription prices. All prices are subject to change without notice. **POSTMASTER:** Send address changes to *Heart Failure Clinics*, Elsevier Health Sciences Division, Subscription Customer Service, 3251 Riverport Lane, Maryland Heights, MO 63043. **Customer Service: 1-800-654-2452 (US and Canada). From outside of the US and Canada, call 314-447-8871. Fax: 314-447-8029. For print support, E-mail: JournalsCustomerService-usa@elsevier.com. For online support, E-mail: JournalsOnlineSupport-usa@elsevier.com.**

Reprints. For copies of 100 or more of articles in this publication, please contact the Commercial Reprints Department, Elsevier Inc., 360 Park Avenue South, New York, NY 10010-1710. Tel.: 212-633-3874; Fax: 212-633-3820; E-mail: reprints@elsevier.com.

Heart Failure Clinics is covered in *MEDLINE/PubMed (Index Medicus)*.

Contributors

CONSULTING EDITORS

MANDEEP R. MEHRA, MD, FACC, FACP, FRCP
Heart and Vascular Center, Brigham and Women's Hospital and Harvard Medical School, Boston, Massachusetts

JAVED BUTLER, MD, MPH, MBA
Stony Brook University Heart Institute, Department of Internal Medicine, Stony Brook School of Medicine, Stony Brook University Medical Center, Stony Brook, New York

EDITORS

PABLO F. CASTRO, MD
Full Professor, Division of Cardiovascular Diseases, Advanced Center for Chronic Diseases FONDAP ACCDis, Facultad de Medicina, Pontificia Universidad Catolica de Chile, Santiago, Chile

NAOKI SATO, MD, PhD, FESC
Cardiology and Intensive Care Unit, Nippon Medical School Musashi-Kosugi Hospital, Kawasaki, Kanagawa, Japan

ROBERT J. MENTZ, MD
Division of Cardiology, Assistant Professor of Medicine, Department of Medicine, Duke University Medical Center, Duke Clinical Research Institute; Duke University School of Medicine, Durham, North Carolina

OVIDIU CHIONCEL, MD, PhD, FHFA
Chair of ICCU and Cardiology 1st Department, Institute of Emergency for Cardiovascular Diseases "C.C.Iliescu", University of Medicine Carol Davila, Bucharest, Romania

AUTHORS

LORA ALKHAWAM, MD
Department of Emergency Medicine, Northwestern University Feinberg School of Medicine, Chicago, Illinois

ANDREW P. AMBROSY, MD
Division of Cardiology, Department of Medicine, Duke University Medical Center, Duke University School of Medicine, Durham, North Carolina

AEKARACH ARIYACHAIPANICH, MD
Excellent Center for Organ Transplantation, King Chulalongkorn Memorial Hospital, Thai Red Cross Society; Division of Cardiology, Department of Medicine, Chulalongkorn University, Bangkok, Thailand

VASILIKI BISTOLA, MD
Heart Failure Unit, Attikon University Hospital, Athens, Greece

JONATHAN BUGGEY, MD
Senior Resident, Department of Medicine, Duke University Medical Center, Duke Medical Hospital, Durham, North Carolina

JUAN F. BULNES, MD
Resident, Division of Internal Medicine, School of Medicine, Pontificia Universidad Catolica de Chile, Santiago, Chile

PABLO F. CASTRO, MD
Full Professor, Division of Cardiovascular Diseases, Advanced Center for Chronic Diseases FONDAP ACCDis, Facultad de Medicina, Pontificia Universidad Catolica de Chile, Santiago, Chile

OVIDIU CHIONCEL, MD, PhD, FHFA
Chair of ICCU and Cardiology 1st Department,
Institute of Emergency for Cardiovascular
Diseases "C.C.Iliescu", University of Medicine
Carol Davila, Bucharest, Romania

MYEONG-CHAN CHO, MD, PhD
Professor, Cardiology Division,
Department of Internal Medicine, College
of Medicine, Chungbuk National
University, Seowon-Gu, Cheongju, Korea

LAUREN B. COOPER, MD
Duke Clinical Research Institute, Durham,
North Carolina

ADAM D. DEVORE, MD
Duke Clinical Research Institute, Durham,
North Carolina

FELIPE DÍAZ-TORO, RN, MPH
Assistant Professor, Facultad de
Enfermería, Escuela de Enfermería,
Universidad Andrés Bello, Santiago,
Chile

G. MICHAEL FELKER, MD, MHS
Duke Clinical Research Institute, Durham,
North Carolina

CATTERINA FERRECCIO, MD, MPH
Full Professor, Advanced Center for
Chronic Diseases FONDAP ACCDis,
Division of Public Health and Family
Medicine, Facultad de Medicina, Pontificia
Universidad Catolica de Chile,
Santiago, Chile

ANTHONY N. GALANOS, MD
Division of Palliative Care, Professor of
Medicine, Department of Medicine, Duke
University Medical Center, Durham, North
Carolina

STEPHEN J. GREENE, MD
Division of Cardiology, Department of
Medicine, Duke University Medical Center;
Duke University School of Medicine, Durham,
North Carolina

DOUGLAS GREIG, MD, MSc
Division of Cardiovascular Diseases,
P Universidad Católica de Chile, Santiago,
Chile

JORGE E. JALIL, MD
Professor of Medicine, Division of
Cardiovascular Diseases, School of Medicine,
Pontificia Universidad Catolica de Chile,
Santiago, Chile

SEOK-MIN KANG, MD, PhD
Cardiology Division, Severance Cardiovascular
Hospital and Cardiovascular Research
Institute, Yonsei University College of
Medicine, Seoul, Korea

SPYRIDON KATSANOS, MD
Heart Failure Unit, Attikon University Hospital,
Athens, Greece

ARUN KRISHNAMOORTHY, MD
Duke University School of Medicine; Duke
Clinical Research Institute, Durham, North
Carolina

**RUNGROJ KRITTAYAPHONG, MD, FACC,
FESC**
Division of Cardiology, Department of
Medicine, Siriraj Hospital, Mahidol University,
Bangkok, Thailand

ALDO PIETRO MAGGIONI, MD, FESC
ANMCO Research Center, Florence, Italy

ALEXANDRE MEBAZAA, MD, FESC, FHFA
Chair of Department of Anesthesia
and Critical Care, Hôpital Lariboisière, DAR,
Hôpitaux Universitaires Saint Louis
Lariboisière, APHP, University Paris Diderot,
Paris, France

ROBERT J. MENTZ, MD
Division of Cardiology, Assistant Professor
of Medicine, Department of Medicine,
Duke University Medical Center, Duke
Clinical Research Institute; Duke
University School of Medicine, Durham,
North Carolina

GABRIEL OLIVARES, MD
Division of Cardiovascular Diseases,
P Universidad Católica de Chile, Santiago,
Chile

JOHN T. PARISSIS, MD
Associate Professor, Heart Failure Unit,
Attikon University Hospital, Athens, Greece

ARTHUR MARK RICHARDS, MBChB, MD, PhD, DSc, FRCP, FRACP, FRSNZ
Professor, Cardiac Department, Director, Cardiovascular Research Institute, National University Heart Centre Singapore, Singapore, Singapore; Department of Medicine, Christchurch Hospital, Director, Christchurch Heart Institute, University of Otago, Christchurch, New Zealand

NAOKI SATO, MD, PhD, FESC
Cardiology and Intensive Care Unit, Nippon Medical School Musashi-Kosugi Hospital, Kawasaki, Kanagawa, Japan

HARRY W. SEVERANCE, MD
Erlanger Institute for Clinical Research, Chattanooga, Tennessee

MUTHIAH VADUGANATHAN, MD, MPH
Heart and Vascular Center, Brigham and Women's Hospital, Boston, Massachusetts

HUGO E. VERDEJO, MD, PhD
Assistant Professor, Division of Cardiovascular Diseases, Advanced Center for Chronic Diseases FONDAP ACCDis, Facultad de Medicina, Pontificia Universidad Catolica de Chile, Santiago, Chile

Contents

Socioeconomic Inequalities in Heart Failure   507

Felipe Díaz-Toro, Hugo E. Verdejo, and Pablo F. Castro

Prevalence and incidence of chronic heart failure (CHF) has increased during the past decades. Beyond its impact on mortality rates, CHF severely impairs quality of life, particularly with the elderly and vulnerable population. Several studies have shown that CHF takes its toll mostly on the uneducated, low-income population, who exhibit impaired access to health care systems, less knowledge regarding its pathology, and poorer self-care behaviors. This review summarizes the available evidence linking socioeconomic inequalities and CHF, focusing on the modifiable factors that may explain the impaired health outcomes in socioeconomically deprived populations.

Heart Failure in Rural Communities   515

Hugo E. Verdejo, Catterina Ferreccio, and Pablo F. Castro

Patients with chronic heart failure (CHF) living in rural areas face an increased risk of adverse cardiovascular events. Even in countries with universal access to health care, rural areas are characteristically underserved, with reduced health care providers supply, greater distance to health care centers, decreased physician density with higher reliance on generalists, and high health care staff turnover. On the other hand, patient-related characteristics vary widely among published data. This review describes the epidemiology of CHF in rural or remote settings, organizational and patient-related factors involved in cardiovascular outcomes, and the role of interventions to improve rural health care.

Inequalities in the Access to Advanced Therapy in Heart Failure   523

Douglas Greig and Gabriel Olivares

At present, heart failure (HF) is a worldwide problem, characterized by a high morbidity and mortality. In industrialized countries or regions, such as the United States, Canada, and western European countries, HF has a prevalence of 1.5% to 2.7%. Chile represents a growing economy in Latin America; however, the relatively high cost of more advanced therapies, in addition to other variables (ie, adequate and timely evaluation by HF specialists), makes access difficult for patients with HF. In this article, the authors review the principal difficulties in accessing advanced HF therapies in Chile, as a model of a developing country.

Gaps and Resemblances in Current Heart Failure Guidelines: A Clinical Perspective   529

Juan F. Bulnes and Jorge E. Jalil

The newly available clinical guidelines in heart failure (HF) from Europe (2012), the United States (2010 and 2013), and Canada (2015) were compared, focusing on the systems for grading the evidence and classifying the recommendations, HF definitions, pharmacologic treatment, and devices used in HF. Some gaps were evident in the methodology for assessing evidence or in HF definitions. Pharmacologic treatments and recommendations for cardiac resynchronization therapy and implantable cardioverter-defibrillators are similar but some differences need to be considered by the practicing clinician. Guideline recommendations regarding new emergent treatments are becoming available.

The hospitalized heart failure (HF) population is becoming a significant economic burden to Asian countries because of the growing elderly population, increased prevalence of HF, and recurrent rehospitalization. A targeted treatment strategy is needed with prognostic factors that can reduce mortality or rehospitalization after discharge. The accepted prognostic factors include age, low systolic blood pressure, ischemic heart disease, reduced left ventricular function, hyponatremia, and renal dysfunction. Prognostic factors for clinical outcomes in hospitalized patients with HF may be different in Asian people. Further research leading to better understanding of the characteristics of Asian patients hospitalized with HF is warranted.

Contributions from the Asian biomedical community to knowledge of biomarkers in heart failure have grown rapidly since 2000. Japan has made world-leading contributions in the discovery and application of cardiac natriuretic peptides as biomarkers in heart failure, but there has been rapid growth in reports from China. Contributions also come from Taiwan, South Korea, Singapore, and Hong Kong. Centers in Asia have established clinical cohorts providing powerful platforms for the discovery and validation of biomarkers in heart failure. This century, Asian enquiry into biomarkers in heart failure will include peptides, cytokines, metabolites, nucleic acids, and other analytes.

The prevalence of heart failure has increased in Asia. A significant proportion of patients with heart failure and left ventricular dysfunction end up with advanced heart failure or end-stage heart disease. These patients may be placed on the waiting list for heart transplant. There are more than 10 countries in Asia that have an active heart transplant program. The number of heart transplants performed is limited despite an increase in the number of patients with end-stage heart failure mainly because of donor shortage, which may be related to religious belief and inefficient allocation policy.

Epidemiologic study is essential to improve management and outcomes in patients hospitalized for heart failure (HF). The academic and socioeconomic status can be clarified by epidemiologic study, and the unsolved issues can be realized. Based on results from epidemiologic studies, strategies to improve the present status could be considered. This article describes several key issues to conduct and interpret an epidemiologic study, for example, definition of HF, time frame, ethnicity, and site selection. Furthermore, assessments and evaluations that are based on comparisons with Western or other Asian data can give a clue to solve the present issues regarding HF management.

Although the prognosis of ambulatory heart failure (HF) has improved dramatically there have been few advances in the management of acute HF (AHF). Despite regional differences in patient characteristics, background therapy, and event rates, AHF clinical trial enrollment has transitioned from North America and Western Europe to Eastern Europe, South America, and Asia-Pacific where regulatory burden and cost of conducting research may be less prohibitive. It is unclear if the results of clinical trials conducted outside of North America are generalizable to US patient populations. This article uses AHF as a paradigm and identifies barriers and practical solutions to successfully conducting site-based research in North America.

Hospitalized heart failure (HHF) patients carry a prognosis comparable to many cancers and constitute more than 1 million hospital admissions annually in the United States. To date, North Americans have comprised a minority of those included in prior hospitalized HF trials and have been repeatedly shown to differ from patients in other areas of the world in terms of clinical characteristics, length of hospital stay, therapy utilization, and post-discharge outcomes. Recognizing the varying patient profiles and outcomes of North Americans enrolled in prior HHF trial programs is critical to optimizing design of future drug development programs and maximizing chances of bringing a novel therapeutic agent to the bedside.

In-hospital worsening heart failure represents a clinical scenario wherein a patient hospitalized for acute heart failure experiences a worsening of their condition, requiring escalation of therapy. Worsening heart failure is associated with worse in-hospital and postdischarge outcomes. Worsening heart failure is increasingly being used as an endpoint or combined endpoint in clinical trials, as it is unique to episodes of acute heart failure and captures an important event during the inpatient course. While prediction models have been developed to identify worsening heart failure, there are no known FDA-approved medications associated with decreased worsening heart failure. Continued study is warranted.

Heart failure (HF) is increasingly common in the United States and is associated with a high degree of morbidity and mortality. As patients approach the end of life there is a significant increase in health care resource use. Patients with end-stage HF have a unique set of needs at the end of life, including symptoms such as dyspnea, uremia, and depression, as well as potentially deactivating implantable defibrillators and mechanical circulatory support devices. Improved palliative care services for patients with HF may improve quality of life and decrease health care resource use near the end of life.

HEART FAILURE CLINICS

ISSUE OF RELATED INTEREST

Cardiology Clinics, February 2014 (Vol. 32, Issue 1)
Heart Failure
Howard J. Eisen, *Editor*
Available at: http://www.cardiology.theclinics.com/

THE CLINICS ARE AVAILABLE ONLINE!
Access your subscription at:
www.theclinics.com

Foreword

Heart Failure: A Global Pandemic and Not Just a Disease of the West

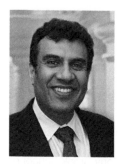   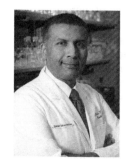

Mandeep R. Mehra, MD, FACC, FACP, FRCP   Javed Butler, MD, MPH, MBA

Consulting Editors

The historic notion that cardiovascular disease, and more specifically heart failure, is a problem of the industrialized western nations, with communicable diseases representing the major source of health problems in the developing nations, is obsolete. Very much like the blurring of the distinction between the "developed" and "developing" nations, differences in population risk factors and disease profiles are also overlapping more in trends between the east and the west. In this respect, there is no doubt that heart failure represents a global pandemic today and poses a serious threat to the health and financial well-being of countries across the globe.

The growing global burden of heart failure represents both the success and failure of the health care system worldwide. In large part, the increasing prevalence of heart failure is related to the aging of the world's population, with higher proportions of elderly in almost all nations and societies. This represents, in part, a failure of the medical system globally, which values and focuses on treatment far in excess of prevention. Despite the growing prevalence of heart failure and its projected worsening epidemiologic trends with the aging population in both the east and the west, efforts to predict risk for heart failure and implementation of interventions for prevention remain in their infancy. Another failure of the health care system that is responsible in part for the global heart failure pandemic is the pervasive suboptimal management of risk factors for cardiovascular disease in patients at high risk (eg, those with hypertension, diabetes mellitus, coronary disease, or obesity). Some of the increased prevalence of heart failure may be attributed to the side-effect profile of effective therapies for other diseases as well (eg, cancer therapy–related cardiac toxicity).

On the other hand, increasing prevalence of heart failure is also a result of the success of the modern practice of medicine, whereby patients with acute and chronic cardiovascular disease, who would have not survived their disease in the past, are now better treated for their cardiovascular diseases (eg, valvular heart disease, myocardial infarction, pulmonary hypertension). Nevertheless, they develop heart failure over time. This trend is likely to be further accentuated as more percutaneous therapies are developed for nonsurgically eligible patients with cardiovascular diseases.

Despite many similarities in etiologies for heart failure, an interesting and important feature of global heart failure burden is regional variability in treatment patterns and outcomes. While some of these may be explained by the differences in the socioeconomic status between regions (eg, the use of implantable automated cardiac defibrillators), other variations are more difficult to explain. For example, the length of stay for acute decompensated heart failure varies widely, with some countries averaging around 4 to 5 days and others 3 to 4 weeks. Such trends may represent, among other reasons, prevalent medical practice cultures between regions.

Heart Failure Clin 11 (2015) xiii–xiv
http://dx.doi.org/10.1016/j.hfc.2015.08.001
1551-7136/15/$ – see front matter © 2015 Published by Elsevier Inc.

It is interesting, however, that even within regions significant variations can be observed. For example, the rate of hospitalization for heart failure varies widely across different regions within the United States. Similarly, within defined geographic regions, significant difference in outcomes has been noted among heart failure patients within racial- and ethnicity-based subgroups. These trends suggest that the outcomes of patients with heart failure depend not only on clinical characteristics or provision of health care but also on nonmedical patient-based variables (eg, socioeconomic, educational, and self-care differences). Such differences and variations in care and outcomes are of concern for clinicians, researchers, and policymakers alike.

Based on these considerations, we invited 4 international experts from North America, South America, Europe, and Asia to assemble a team of experts from around the world to give us a global perspective on heart failure. They cover topics including insights into epidemiology, socioeconomic inequalities, issues pertinent to rural communities, access to care, differences in care, prognosis determination, and outcomes to intensive care, advanced care, and palliative care. We hope that this broad perspective on heart failure will be equally important for clinicians, researchers, and policymakers, and that readers gain granular insights from our team of expert authors and guest editors.

Mandeep R. Mehra, MD, FACC, FACP, FRCP
Heart and Vascular Center
Center for Advanced Heart Disease
Brigham and Women's Hospital
Harvard Medical School
75 Francis Street, A Building
3rd Floor, Room AB324
Boston, MA 02115, USA

Javed Butler, MD, MPH, MBA
Stony Brook University Heart Institute
Department of Internal Medicine
Stony Brook School of Medicine
Stony Brook University Medical Center
101 Nicolls Road
Stony Brook, NY 11794, USA

E-mail addresses:
MMEHRA@partners.org (M.R. Mehra)
Javed.Butler@stonybrookmedicine.edu (J. Butler)

Socioeconomic Inequalities in Heart Failure

Felipe Díaz-Toro, RN, MPH[a],*, Hugo E. Verdejo, MD, PhD[b],
Pablo F. Castro, MD[b]

KEYWORDS

- Heart failure • Socioeconomic status • Health care disparities • Health literacy

KEY POINTS

- Socioeconomic inequalities directly influence the incidence, management, and prognosis of patients with chronic heart failure (CHF).
- Socioeconomic status (SES) is a powerful independent predictor of CHF development and adverse outcomes. Low SES is associated with reduced access to care, decreased levels of knowledge, and reduced health literacy.
- Limited health literacy is associated with decreased knowledge about medical condition, poor medication recall, nonadherence to treatment plans, poor self-care behaviors, poorer physical and mental health, increased hospitalizations, and increased mortality.

BACKGROUND

Chronic heart failure (CHF) is defined as a functional or structural abnormality in the heart that impairs ventricular filling or ventricular ejection fraction, causing a mismatch between oxygen supply and metabolic requirements of peripheral tissues. CHF is a complex clinical syndrome representing the end stage of several cardiovascular pathologies and is characterized by typical signs and symptoms, such as dyspnea, peripheral edema, intolerance to exertion, and pulmonary congestion.[1,2]

Prevalence of CHF has systematically increased during the past decades.[2] Demographic changes due to an aging population, an increase in cardiovascular risk factors, and advances in pharmacologic therapy may explain the growing number of patients with CHF. In the United States, the estimated prevalence of CHF is 5.8 million cases and constitutes the first cause of hospitalization in elderly patients.[3]

In general terms, between 1% and 2% of the adult population of developed countries have CHF. The prevalence markedly increases with age, reaching as high as 10% for patients aged 70 years or older. Data on CHF incidence is scarce, but a conservative estimate of 5 to 10 per 1000 persons per year translates to 550,000 new cases of CHF each year in the United States alone.[3,4] The World Health Organization puts CHF within the 5 leading causes of death in adults worldwide. If the current epidemic growth of CHF does not change, by 2030 more than 8,000,000 deaths worldwide of the population aged 30 years or older will be caused by CHF.[5]

The impact of CHF on public health goes beyond its growing incidence and prevalence. Health costs

Disclosure statement: The author has nothing to disclose.
[a] Facultad de Enfermería, Escuela de Enfermería, Universidad Andrés Bello, Sazié 2212, 6th Floor, Santiago 8370136, Chile; [b] Advanced Center for Chronic Diseases, Escuela de Medicina, Pontificia Universidad Catolica de Chile, Santiago 8330024, Chile
* Corresponding author.
E-mail address: felipe.diaz.t@unab.cl

Heart Failure Clin 11 (2015) 507–513
http://dx.doi.org/10.1016/j.hfc.2015.07.012

related to CHF put a considerable stress on health care systems, mainly due to repeated visits to emergency rooms and repeated hospitalizations.[4,6,7] At the same time, patients with CHF exhibit a severely impaired quality of life, which further deteriorates after each rehospitalization.[8] Several studies have shown that CHF predominantly affects lower-income, poorly educated people. More educated, higher-income people usually report lower morbidity from common chronic diseases (stroke, hypertension, dyslipidemia, diabetes). Physical and mental functioning is also better for the better educated; they are substantially less likely to report that they are in poor health, and less likely to report anxiety or depression.[9–12]

Socioeconomic status (SES) is a complex, multidimensional concept that involves several determinants of health. Several indicators have been used as surrogate markers for SES; their relative importance varies during different stages of the life course. Common indicators for SES are educational level, income, self-perceived social class, housing characteristics, employment relations, and health literacy, among others.[12] In developed countries, educational level, employment relations, and household income are strong predictors for death or rehospitalization in patients with cardiovascular diseases (CVD). However, their association with CHF is less certain.[13,14]

Most of these indicators evidence the underlying inequalities that link SES to health outcomes. Poorer, uneducated patients have less access to appropriate health care, and may not be able to understand the key information to establish self-care behaviors. The concept of health literacy comprises the abilities, knowledge, and management capacities of an individual regarding their pathology. Patients with low literacy often exhibit nonadherent behaviors and low use of preventive care with a higher number of visits to emergency rooms and an increased rate of rehospitalization.[9,15]

This review aims to assess the impact of SES inequities on CHF, focusing on the effect of income, education, and health literacy in CHF outcomes.

SOCIOECONOMIC STATUS AND HEART FAILURE

The association between low SES and coronary artery disease (CAD) is well known; however, the relationship between CHF and socioeconomic deprivation is far less understood. Low SES increases the risk of both CAD and CHF[16]; however, whether this reflects a direct association of SES and CHF or an indirect effect is not known. Both CAD and CHF share common risk factors; in fact, nearly 50% of patients with CAD will develop

CHF.[12] Lower SES also relates to higher prevalence of type 2 diabetes in the middle years of life,[17] as well as hypertension.[18] These findings suggest that exposure to factors implicated in the causation of CVD, and ultimately CHF, is more common in deprived areas. This may explain the effect of low education level, which precedes the onset of most behaviors associated with increased CVD. Elementary school education is associated with increased risk of CHF in a representative US population sample with a population attributable risk of 9%.[16]

A recently published systematic review including 28 studies aimed to elucidate the association between CHF and SES. Main outcomes were incidence, prevalence, hospitalizations, mortality, and treatment of CHF. Socioeconomic measures included education, occupation, employment relations, social class, income, housing characteristics, and composite and area-level indicators. Lower SES was associated with increased incidence of CHF, either in the community or of people presenting to the hospital. The adjusted risk of developing CHF was increased by 30% to 50% in most reports for patients with lower SES. Readmission rates following hospitalization were likewise greater in more deprived patients. Although fewer studies examined mortality, lower SES was associated with poorer survival. The investigators concluded that "socioeconomic deprivation is a powerful independent predictor of heart failure development and adverse outcomes."[12]

EDUCATIONAL LEVEL AND OCCUPATION

Several studies have evaluated the association between CHF and educational level. Christensen and colleagues[19] followed a prospective cohort of 2190 patients from the Copenhagen City Heart Study, hospitalized for CHF. In this cohort, intermediate (8–10 years of education) and higher education (>10 years) were associated with an important decrease in the risk of CHF development (relative ratio [RR] 0.69, 95% confidence interval [CI] 0.62–0.78 and 0.52, 95% CI 0.43–0.63, respectively).

Similar findings were reported by He and colleagues[16] in the National Health and Nutrition Examination Survey I cohort. This study followed 13,000 subjects without CHF for 19 years. During the follow-up, 1400 patients were diagnosed and hospitalized due to CHF. Less than high school education conveyed an increased risk for hospital admission or death from CHF after a multivariable adjustment (RR 1.22, 95% CI 1.04–1.42; $P = .01$). In Sweden, Ingelsson and colleagues[20] followed a cohort of men aged 50 years or older. Among these subjects, those with a lower educational level had an increased risk for CHF development when compared with those of higher education, even after adjustment for hypertension, diabetes, electrocardiographic left ventricular hypertrophy, smoking, serum cholesterol, and interim myocardial infarction (hazard ratio [HR] 1.98, 95% CI 1.07–3.68).

Benderly and colleagues[21] followed 2951 subjects free from CHF included in the BIP cohort (Bezafibrate Infarction Prevention) for a mean of 8 years. During this period, 511 patients developed CHF. Patients who developed CHF were less educated, with 44% having only elementary education compared with 36% of patients without HF, and 15% with an academic education versus 19% of patients free of HF. Similarly, academic or higher occupations were reported for 28% of patients who developed HF compared with 41% of patients who did not.

Using data from the British Regional Heart Study, Ramsay and colleagues[22] followed a cohort of 3836 men between 60 and 79 years old for a period of 10 years. During follow-ups, 229 subjects developed CHF. Consistent with previous results, adult socioeconomic position (based on a cumulative score, including occupation, education, housing tenure, pension, and amenities) predicted the development of CHF even after adjustment for systolic blood pressure, body mass index, smoking, high-density lipoprotein cholesterol, diabetes, and lung function. The effect of socioeconomic deprivation on CHF was only partly explained by established risk factors for HF (1.87, 95% CI 1.12–3.11).

In an attempt to evaluate the association of occupation and CHF, Schaufelberger and Rosengren[11] analyzed data derived from participant men from the intervention group in the multifactor Primary Prevention Study that began in Göteborg, Sweden, in 1970. Of the 1004 subjects whose discharge diagnosis or cause of death was HF, subjects in a lower occupational class had higher risk for CHF, with a 72% increased risk in unskilled workers compared with high officials. Compared with the highest occupational class, unskilled workers had an age-adjusted HR of 1.92 (95% CI 1.50–2.45) of developing CHF. Semiskilled and skilled workers (HR 1.59, 95% CI 1.25–2.03) and lower officials and foremen (HR 1.62, 95% CI 1.26–2.10) had intermediate risks.

In Latin America, the information regarding CHF and SES is scarce, but the few published series are consistent with previously published results. In Chile, results from the National Registry of Heart Failure (ICARO) show that lower educational level was associated with increased prevalence of CHF. From a total of 370 patients admitted due to decompensated CHF, 61% had basic education, 17% had intermediate-high education, and 9% were illiterate.[23] The same group published the results of 900 patients followed during 10 years. In this cohort, all-cause mortality was 20% higher in patients with lower SES and CHF.[24]

Other Latin American countries, such as Brazil and Argentina, have acknowledged the social problem stemming from the association of socioeconomic inequalities and increased risk of CVD. Lower SES is associated with higher CVD disease in Buenos Aires, Argentina,[25] as well as in some urban regions in Brazil.[26] Even when health care reforms have translated to better access to health in most Latin American countries, the effect of socioeconomic inequalities persists. Furthermore, mortality for CVD has decreased more rapidly in high-affluence, higher-education areas in Sao Paulo.[27]

HEALTH LITERACY AND HEART FAILURE

An emerging indicator of health inequalities is health literacy, defined as "the degree to which individuals have the capacity to obtain, process, and understand basic health information and services needed to make appropriate health decisions."[9,10] This definition goes beyond the ability to read and understand a text provided by health care personnel. It incorporates the ability to understand complex vocabulary, share information with health care professionals, make decisions regarding healthy behaviors, and participate actively in the management and self-care of chronic diseases.[15]

Several tools have been designed to assess health literacy. The more commonly used in epidemiologic studies are summarized on **Table 1**.

The impact of health literacy in CHF is multidimensional. Patients with low health literacy may have problems managing their disease due to lack of understanding of indications from health caregivers regarding pharmacologic treatment and lifestyle modification. Low health literacy directly impairs the ability to acquire knowledge regarding their disease, decreasing therapeutic adherence as well as the chances to establish self-care behaviors. Patients with low health literacy do not use preventive health services correctly, have bad mental and physical health, and exhibit an increased mortality risk and increased rate of hospitalization due to decompensated CHF when compared with the high health literacy population.[9,15,34]

DeWalt and colleagues[35] conducted a meta-analysis including articles published between 1980 and 2003 across 17 databases, and concluded that low literacy is associated with several adverse health outcomes, including increased risk of

Table 1
Instruments to assess health literacy

Tool Acronym	Full Name	Time to Administer, min
NVS	Newest Vital Sign[28]	3
SILS	Single Item Literacy Screener[29]	<1
REALM	Rapid Estimate of Adult Literacy in Medicine[30]	2–3
REALM-R	Rapid Estimate of Adult Literacy in Medicine (Revised) (Medical Word recognition test)[30]	2–3
WRAT-R	Wide Range Achievement Test Revised[30]	3–8
(S) TOFHLA	Test of Functional Health Literacy in Adults[31] (S) = Short Version[32]	Short: 7 Long: 22
SAHLSA	Short Assessment of Health Literacy for Spanish Speaking Adults[33]	5

hospitalization and lack of knowledge about health services. A recently published systematic review by Cajita and colleagues[9] included 23 studies encompassing 11,200 patients with CHF. On average, 39% of the patients with CHF had low literacy. Older patients had less knowledge about their disease, even after adjustment by educational level, race, gender, and immigration status. Women had higher levels of health literacy after adjustment by age, race, education, income, sensory function, and cognitive function. As was expected, educational level was positively related to health literacy (odds ratio [OR] 5.04; 95% CI 3.31–7.69; P<.001), as well as cognitive function (r = 0.545; P<.01). African Americans had lower levels of health literacy even after adjustment for confounding variables. Low health literacy was found to be associated with increased incidence of CHF-related hospitalizations (incident rate ratio (IRR) 1.42, 95% CI 1.11–1.83) even after controlling for age, race, gender, SES, educational level, insurance coverage, clinical characteristics, and self-management skills.

Wu and colleagues[34] showed that in a cohort of 595 patients with CHF, low literacy predicts a higher risk for death or hospitalization. Individuals with low literacy had an IRR of 1.39 (95% CI 0.99–1.94) for all-cause hospitalization or death and 1.36 (1.11–1.66) for HF-related hospitalization. After adjusting for demographic, clinical, and self management factors, the IRRs were 1.31 (1.06–1.63) for all-cause hospitalization and death, and 1.46 (1.20–1.78) for HF-related hospitalization. Similarly, McNaughton and colleagues[36] showed in a cohort of 1379 subjects an increased HR for death among patients with low health literacy (HR 1.34, 95% CI 1.04–1.73, P = .02).

Similar results showed Peterson and colleagues[37] in a cohort of 1547 patients with diagnosis of CHF. On average, 17.5% had low health

literacy. Patients with low health literacy were older, socially deprived, less educated, and with more comorbidities than other subjects. Low health literacy was an independent mortality predictor, the unadjusted rate was 17.6% versus 6.3% (adjusted HR 1.97 (95% CI 1.3–2.97); P = .001). Moser and colleagues[38] examined the association of health literacy with heart failure in those living in rural areas. A sample of 575 patients hospitalized for heart failure within the past 6 months and followed for 2 years, showed that 19.1% of patients were characterized with inadequate health literacy, 16.7% in the marginal category and 64.2% with adequate health literacy. The patients with low health literacy were older, male, less educated, and unemployed. Unadjusted analysis revealed that patients with inadequate or marginal health literacy were 1.94 (95% CI 1.43–2.63, P<.001) times and 1.91 (95% CI 1.36–2.67, P<.001) times, respectively, for rehospitalizations or all-cause mortality.

BRIDGING THE GAPS IN SOCIOECONOMIC INEQUALITY

Components of SES, such as level of education, income, or occupation are hard to modify; any effort aimed at correcting them on a population basis implies the development of public policies, with a considerable expense of economic and human resources. A much more efficient use of public resources is to design and implement prevention strategies aimed at correcting easily modifiable risk factors that have a larger impact on CVD risk. Hence, health policy makers have advocated for programs focused on promoting healthy lifestyles and modifying risk-related behaviors through education and counseling as the pillars for community-wide health promotion. In the particular case of CHF, even when knowledge about the disease is insufficient by itself to improve therapeutic adherence, it is the minimal requirement to promote behavioral changes associated with self-care.[39]

Boyde and colleagues[40] published a meta-analysis of educational interventions in CHF including 19 randomized controlled trials from 1998 to 2008 (2686 patients). The usual educational intervention was a one-on-one nurse-led session supplemented by written materials and multimedia approaches. Even when educational programs alone improved knowledge levels, the interventions had a variable effect on outcomes. Interestingly, although most trials involved nurse-led patient education, the scope of educational programs may involve the whole community. In Iran, Siabani and colleagues[41] showed that a home-based, face-to-face education program provided by community volunteers improved self-care maintenance and self-care management in patients with CHF as effectively as the education provided by health professionals in a formal health education program, and much better than the usual care. When education is incorporated in a comprehensive disease-management or tele-health program, more robust results are reported, such as reduction of disease-related hospital admissions, mortality, and improved health-related quality of life.[42]

Less is known regarding the role of health literacy in CHF. Expert guided recommendations to increase patient literacy suggest a stepwise approach, assisting the patient in recognizing that there is a problem and afterward engaging in a respectful assessment of the individual's needs, skills, and competencies. Interventions aimed to increase literacy and improve communication between patients and health care providers, encourages patients to become active members of their health care team. However, the impact of these recommendations on the design of interventions aimed at health literacy as a tool to promote improved health outcomes is still largely unknown.[43]

FUTURE DIRECTIONS

The association between socioeconomic inequality and CVD risk factors has been extensively studied, but several aspects remain uncertain. In particular, the association between CHF and SES is still a controversial issue, with many investigators attributing it to the effect of confounding variables, such as increased morbidity and impaired access to care. To elucidate this relationship, future studies with large population cohorts at diverse life stages will be required to assess whether healthy life habits and improved education have a positive impact on CHF lifetime prevalence. The promise of education for patients with CHF as a tool to reduce hospitalizations and death has yet to be realized. Despite improvements in knowledge, outcome results are variable and likely depend on the type of intervention and the existence of an organized CHF management program. There is a growing amount of evidence that patient health literacy is critical to translate any educational intervention to self-care behaviors. Knowledge about health literacy and CHF is still in an early stage. Studies aimed at characterizing the clinical and socioeconomic profile of patients with CHF with low literacy are urgently needed to implement an effective patient-centered educational approach in CHF.

SUMMARY

Socioeconomic inequalities directly influence the incidence, management, and prognosis of patients with CHF. Several studies have shown that surrogate markers of SES, such as level of education, occupation, and income are independent predictors of rehospitalization and mortality, even after adjustment for comorbidities, age, and gender. These findings explain why even in universal access health systems, with well-developed outpatient support, rehospitalization for decompensated CHF remains a major cause for hospital admission. Low-health literacy provides a reliable estimation of the disease management abilities in an outpatient setting. In contrast with other SES markers, health literacy is a modifiable risk factor; interventions aimed to increase disease awareness and disease-related knowledge may foster the development of self-care behaviors, reducing the risk of rehospitalization and ultimately improving event-free survival and quality of life in patients with CHF.

REFERENCES

1. McMurray JJ, Adamopoulos S, Anker SD, et al. ESC guidelines for the diagnosis and treatment of acute and chronic heart failure 2012: the task force for the diagnosis and treatment of acute and chronic heart failure 2012 of the European Society of Cardiology. Developed in collaboration with the Heart Failure Association (HFA) of the ESC. Eur Heart J 2012;33: 1787–847.
2. Yancy CW, Jessup M, Bozkurt B, et al. ACCF/AHA guideline for the management of heart failure: a report of the American College of Cardiology Foundation/American Heart Association Task Force on Practice Guidelines. J Am Coll Cardiol 2013;62: e147–239.

3. Roger VL, Weston SA, Redfield MM, et al. Trends in heart failure incidence and survival in a community-based population. JAMA 2004;292:344–50.

4. Roger VL. Epidemiology of heart failure. Circ Res 2013;113:646–59.

5. Bloom DE, Cafiero ET, Jané-Llopis E, et al. The global economic burden of noncommunicable diseases. Geneva (Switzerland): World Economic Forum; 2010.

6. Bocchi EA, Arias A, Verdejo H, et al. The reality of heart failure in Latin America. J Am Coll Cardiol 2013;62:949–58.

7. Bui AL, Horwich TB, Fonarow GC. Epidemiology and risk profile of heart failure. Nat Rev Cardiol 2010;8: 30–41.

8. Nieminen MS, Dickstein K, Fonseca C, et al. The patient perspective: quality of life in advanced heart failure with frequent hospitalisations. Int J Cardiol 2015;191:256–64.

9. Cajita MI, Cajita TR, Han H-R. Health literacy and heart failure. J Cardiovasc Nurs 2015. [Epub ahead of print].

10. Robinson S, Moser D, Pelter MM, et al. Assessing health literacy in heart failure patients. J Card Fail 2011;17:887–92.

11. Schaufelberger M, Rosengren A. Heart failure in different occupational classes in Sweden. Eur Heart J 2006;28:212–8.

12. Hawkins NM, Jhund PS, McMurray JJV, et al. Heart failure and socioeconomic status: accumulating evidence of inequality. Eur J Heart Fail 2014;14: 138–46.

13. Mackenbach J. Socioeconomic inequalities in cardiovascular disease mortality. An international study. Eur Heart J 2000;21:1141–51.

14. Cleland J. The EuroHeart Failure survey programme—a survey on the quality of care among patients with heart failure in Europe Part 1: patient characteristics and diagnosis. Eur Heart J 2003;24: 442–63.

15. Evangelista L, Rasmusson K, Laramee A, et al. Health literacy and the patient with heart failure—implications for patient care and research: a consensus statement of the Heart Failure Society of America. J Card Fail 2010;16:9–16.

16. He J, Ogden LG, Bazzano LA, et al. Risk factors for congestive heart failure in US men and women: NHANES I epidemiologic follow-up study. Arch Intern Med 2001;161:996–1002.

17. Connolly V, Unwin N, Sherriff P, et al. Diabetes prevalence and socioeconomic status: a population based study showing increased prevalence of type 2 diabetes mellitus in deprived areas. J Epidemiol Community Health 2000;54:173–7.

18. Colhoun HM, Hemingway H. Socio-economic status and blood pressure: an overview analysis. J Hum Hypertens 1998;12:91–110.

19. Christensen S, Mogelvang R, Heitmann M, et al. Level of education and risk of heart failure: a prospective cohort study with echocardiography evaluation. Eur Heart J 2011;32:450–8.

20. Ingelsson E, Lind L, Arnlöv J, et al. Socioeconomic factors as predictors of incident heart failure. J Card Fail 2006;12:540–5.

21. Benderly M, Haim M, Boyko V, et al. Socioeconomic status indicators and incidence of heart failure among men and women with coronary heart disease. J Card Fail 2013;19:117–24.

22. Ramsay SE, Whincup PH, Papacosta O, et al. Inequalities in heart failure in older men: prospective associations between socioeconomic measures and heart failure incidence in a 10-year follow-up study. Eur Heart J 2014;35:442–7.

23. Vukasovic JL, Castro P, Sepúlveda L, et al. Insuficiencia cardíaca en hospitales chilenos: resultados del Registro Nacional de Insuficiencia Cardíaca, Grupo ICARO. Rev Med Chil 2006;134:539–48.

24. Castro P, Verdejo H, Garcés E, et al. Influencia de factores socioculturales en la evolución alejada de pacientes con insuficiencia cardíaca. Rev Chil Cardiol 2009;28:51–62.

25. Diez Roux AV, Green Franklin T, Alazraqui M, et al. Intraurban variations in adult mortality in a large Latin American city. J Urban Health 2007;84: 319–33.

26. Nogueira M, Ribeiro L, Cruz O. Desigualdades sociais na mortalidade cardiovascular precoce em um município de médio porte no Brasil. Cad Saude Pública 2009;25(11):2321–32 [cited 2015-06-01].

27. Soares GP, Brum JD, Oliveira G. Evolution of socioeconomic indicators and cardiovascular mortality in three Brazilian states. Arq Bras Cardiol 2013;100(2): 147–56.

28. Weiss BD, Mays MZ, Martz W, et al. Quick assessment of literacy in primary care: the newest vital sign. Ann Fam Med 2005;3:514–22.

29. Davis TC, Long SW, Jackson RH, et al. Rapid estimate of adult literacy in medicine: a shortened screening instrument. Fam Med 1993;25:391–5.

30. Bass PF, Wilson JF, Griffith CH. A shortened instrument for literacy screening. J Gen Intern Med 2003;18:1036–8.

31. Parker RM, Baker DW, Williams MV, et al. The test of functional health literacy in adults: a new instrument for measuring patients' literacy skills. J Gen Intern Med 1995;10:537–41.

32. Baker DW, Williams MV, Parker RM, et al. Development of a brief test to measure functional health literacy. Patient Educ Couns 1999;38:33–42.

33. Lee S-YD, Bender DE, Ruiz RE, et al. Development of an easy-to-use Spanish Health Literacy test. Health Serv Res 2006;41:1392–412.

34. Wu J-R, Holmes GM, DeWalt DA, et al. Low literacy is associated with increased risk of hospitalization

and death among individuals with heart failure. J Gen Intern Med 2013;28:1174–80.

35. DeWalt DA, Berkman ND, Sheridan S. Literacy and health outcomes. J Gen Intern Med 2004;19(12): 1228–39.

36. McNaughton CD, Cawthon C, Kripalani S, et al. Health literacy and mortality: a cohort study of patients hospitalized for acute heart failure. J Am Heart Assoc 2015;4:e001799.

37. Peterson PN, Shetterly SM, Clarke CL, et al. Health literacy and outcomes among patients with heart failure. JAMA 2011;305:1695–701.

38. Moser DK, Robinson S, Biddle MJ, et al. Health literacy predicts morbidity and mortality in rural patients with heart failure. J Card Fail 2015. [Epub ahead of print].

39. Lainscak M, Blue L, Clark AL, et al. Self-care management of heart failure: practical recommendations from the Patient Care Committee of the Heart Failure

Association of the European Society of Cardiology. Eur J Heart Fail 2011;13:115–26.

40. Boyde M, Turner C, Thompson DR, et al. Educational interventions for patients with heart failure: a systematic review of randomized controlled trials. J Cardiovasc Nurs 2011;26:E27–35.

41. Siabani S, Driscoll T, Davidson PM, et al. Efficacy of a home-based educational strategy involving community health volunteers in improving self-care in patients with chronic heart failure in western Iran: a randomized controlled trial. Eur J Cardiovasc Nurs 2015 [pii:1474515115585651].

42. Bos-Touwen I, Jonkman N, Westland H, et al. Tailoring of self-management interventions in patients with heart failure. Curr Heart Fail Rep 2015; 12:223–35.

43. Westlake C, Sethares K, Davidson P. How can health literacy influence outcomes in heart failure patients? Mechanisms and interventions. Curr Heart Fail Rep 2013;10:232–43.

Heart Failure in Rural Communities

Hugo E. Verdejo, MD, PhD[a],*, Catterina Ferreccio, MD, MPH[b], Pablo F. Castro, MD[a]

KEYWORDS

- Rural health • Heart failure • Health care disparities

KEY POINTS

- Living in a rural setting has been associated with poorer health and decreased consumption of health care.
- Organizational elements, such as decreased health care providers supply, longer distance to health care centers, and low density of physicians, may contribute to adverse outcomes of chronic heart failure (CHF) in rural communities.
- Rural patients with CHF are slower to adopt healthy behaviors and have lower levels of health literacy when compared with urban patients with CHF. Interventions aimed to increase disease-related knowledge in patients with CHF may have a favorable impact on rehospitalization and quality of life.
- The challenge to improve rural CHF management involves multidisciplinary support to optimize CHF diagnosis, use of new monitoring technologies, improved therapeutic guideline adherence, and optimized outpatient self-management.

BACKGROUND

During the past century, industrialized societies underwent a major epidemiologic transition characterized by a shift of the main causes of death from infectious disease and nutritional deficiencies to more chronic, nontransmissible diseases, such as cardiovascular disease.[1] On the other hand, lower-income economies underwent an asymmetrical process characterized by progressive urbanization of large cities, rural-urban migration as a response to the perceived inequalities in wealth, and increased rural resource scarcity (**Box 1**).[2]

Today, urban communities have a higher risk-factor burden than rural communities but, nevertheless, exhibit a lower rate of adverse cardiovascular events. The Prospective Urban Rural Epidemiology (PURE) trial included 156,424 persons from 348 urban and 280 rural communities on 5 continents who were followed up for a mean of 4.1 years. Rates of all cardiovascular events as well as fatal cardiovascular events were higher in rural communities (4.83 vs 6.25 events per 1000 persons-years, $P<.001$ and 1.71 vs 3.09 events per 1000 person-years, $P<.01$, respectively). The INTERHEART risk score was higher in rural areas in high-income countries (13.43 vs 12.67, $P<.01$), but the inverse tendency was observed in middle- and low-income areas (10.11 vs 10.81, $P<.001$ and 7.57 vs 9.09, $P<.001$, respectively).[3] These disparate results (lower risk profile but higher cardiovascular mortality) suggest that health determinants other than those included in traditional risk-factor assessments are responsible in the adverse health outcomes observed in rural communities.

Disclosure statement: The authors have nothing to disclose.
[a] Division of Cardiovascular Diseases, Advanced Center for Chronic Diseases FONDAP ACCDis, Facultad de Medicina, Pontificia Universidad Catolica de Chile, Marcoleta 367, CP 8330024, Santiago, Chile; [b] Advanced Center for Chronic Diseases FONDAP ACCDis, Division of Public Health and Family Medicine, Facultad de Medicina, Pontificia Universidad Catolica de Chile, Marcoleta 434, CP 8330073, Santiago, Chile
* Corresponding author. Division of Cardiovascular Diseases, Marcoleta 367 8vo Piso, Santiago, Chile.
E-mail address: hverdejo@med.puc.cl

heartfailure.theclinics.com

Box 1
What does rural mean?

- The word *rural* is often associated with agricultural communities with low population density and variable degrees of geographic isolation. However, the operative definition of rural varies widely depending on the source and purpose.

- The US Office of Management and Budget defines a county as a metropolitan statistical area (MSA) if it contains an urban core of greater than 50,000 individuals. Any county that does not fulfill this characteristic is considered rural. Non-MSA counties can be further categorized into micropolitan (those with an urban core between 10,000 and 50,000 inhabitants) and noncore counties.

- The US Census Bureau defines urbanized areas as those with population cores of 50,000 or more inhabitants. Urban clusters have cores between 2500 and 50,000 inhabitants. All other areas are designated rural.

- The Organization for Economic Cooperation and Development defines a rural community as any local administrative unit level 2 with a population density less than 150 inhabitants per square kilometer. A predominantly rural region is a geographic area in which more than 50% of the inhabitants live in a rural community

- In India, the National Institute for Rural Development defines rural sector as any place as per the latest available census that has a population of less than 5,000, with a population density of less than 400 inhabitants per square kilometer and in which more than 25% of the male working population is engaged in agricultural pursuits.

EPIDEMIOLOGY

Traditionally, living in a rural setting has been associated with poorer health[4] and decreased consumption of health care.[5] This concern is not new; in 1966, Gibson and colleagues[6] published a first attempt to characterize chronic heart failure (CHF) epidemiology in 2 rural communities from North Carolina and Vermont and reported an increased prevalence of CHF (8.8 and 10.2 cases per 1000 habitants). The current evidence regarding the prevalence of CHF in rural versus urban communities is controversial and may exhibit considerable variation between countries. Clark and colleagues[7] performed a cross-sectional survey that included 23,845 subjects in Australia. The survey revealed a significantly higher prevalence of CHF among general practice patients in large and small rural towns (16.1%) compared with capital city and metropolitan areas (12.4%) ($P<.001$). Conversely, Yang and colleagues[8] reported a decreased prevalence in rural China using a self-reported questionnaire (1.1% vs 0.8%). The epidemiology of CHF in rural communities from other developing countries is very poorly established; for most countries, there are no published data and the available registries include hospital-based series subject to substantial selection bias.[9,10]

Even when the absolute prevalence of CHF in rural settings may seem controversial, most investigators agree that rural areas has a 1.5 higher rate of potentially preventable hospitalizations caused by chronic diseases, such as CHF; this risk has increased in the last decade despite a decline in

the rate of admissions for remote rural areas.[11] This issue is also controversial, as small studies had reported a decreased rate of rehospitalization for rural patients with CHF. However, the appropriateness of this end point when assessing CHF outpatient outcomes is dubious. For instance, Wu and colleagues[12] reported a better event-free survival in rural patients with CHF using the composite end point of emergency department (ED) visits and rehospitalization; but the study was underpowered to detect a difference in death rates, and it did not account for access to health care facilities.

Several factors may influence this outcome: health care providers supply, population health literacy, distance to health care centers, increasing reliance on generalists, and so forth.[5] These factors, however, may not be consistent in all settings. Harris and colleagues[13] showed that hospitalization rates in Maine depend mainly on confounding variables, such as unemployment and poverty. Neither rurality nor physician density influenced hospitalization rates in this particular setting.

Increased prevalence and higher risk for hospitalizations contribute heavily to the increased mortality associated with heart failure in rural settings but do not fully explain the observed differences with urban patients with CHF. Several studies have tried to elucidate the causes underlying the more adverse health results in rural communities. Teng and colleagues[14] analyzed a large cohort of 17,379 Australian patients after a first CHF hospitalization. Rural patients (25.9%) were significantly younger, without significant differences in the prevalence of coronary artery disease (CAD), hypertension, or diabetes mellitus. After adjusting for age, rural patients had higher 30-day and 1-year mortality after discharge (odds ratio [OR] 1.16, 95% confidence interval [CI] 1.01–1.33 and hazard ratio [HR] 1.11, 95% CI 1.01–1.23, respectively). Interestingly, this difference persisted even when socioeconomic status, emergency presentation, and aboriginality were included in the model, suggesting the participation of other variables in the observed geographic variation. One possible explanation was the type of care received by patients with CHF; around 75% of the rural patients were managed in small district hospitals, whereas the most urban patients were managed in tertiary centers. Similar imbalances in health care access and utilization between urban and rural communities have already been identified in North America,[15,16] Asia,[17] and Latin America.[10,18,19]

ORGANIZATIONAL FACTORS IN RURAL HEALTH SYSTEMS
Health System Policies

Hospitalizations caused by decompensated CHF are considered ambulatory-care sensitive hospitalizations based on the concept that they might be avoided by the timely provision of out-of-hospital care to prevent exacerbations. In the United States, potentially preventable hospitalizations account for nearly 10% of all hospitalizations. In 2005, rural areas had a 49.9% higher rate of potentially preventable hospitalizations; by 2011, this prevalence increased to 57.2%.[11]

Although programs for CHF management exist in most countries, ensuring universal access remains a challenge. Optimal treatment of CHF involves evidence-based, multidisciplinary, patient-centered care. In rural settings, the combination of limited resource availability, initial diagnostic delay, suboptimal management, and lack of an integrated clinical information system contribute to the decreased access to healthcare.[20] A regression analysis based on nationwide data from Germany, in 2008, showed that an increase in the density of the practice of general practitioners by 1 per 100,000 inhabitants was associated with an absolute reduction in 0.1% in the rate of hospitalizations caused by decompensated CHF.[21] Special admission programs, such as the Physicians for Shortage Area Program of Jefferson Medical College, have increased the percentage of rural family physicians; increased the retaining of physicians in rural health care; and, despite its small size, showed a major impact on the rural physician workforce, accounting for 21% of rural family physicians in Pennsylvania.[22]

The impact of practitioner density may particularly impact the ability to provide a proper ambulatory management. For instance, early physician follow-up (within 7 days after discharge) is critical to reduce 30-day readmission rates in patients with CHF,[23] particularly in elderly rural patients.[24] In a cohort of 30,160 patients from the Organized Program to Initiate Lifesaving Treatment in Hospitalized Patients With Heart Failure (OPTIMIZE) and Get with the Guidelines-Heart Failure (GWTG-HF) registries, 37.9% patients had early physician follow-up, in stark contrast with the rate of early physician control in rural communities of 17% (OR 0.84, CI 95% 0.78–0.91); conversely, higher physician density increased the odds of early follow-up. These associations persisted even after modifying the definition of early follow-up to 14 days after discharge.[25] Even in systems with universal access to care in which the total number of physician encounters after discharge is similar for urban and rural patients with CHF, there is an increase in the number of events in rural populations that implies different models of care between urban and rural centers. In urban centers, patients are more likely to be seen in physician offices, decreasing the number of visits to EDs.[15]

In an effort to provide appropriate health care to rural areas, the Medicare Rural Hospital Flexibility program created the designation of critical access hospitals (CAH) to small, isolated hospitals with less than 25 acute care beds and separated more than 35 miles to the nearest hospital. In a survey of 4738 US hospitals, CAHs exhibited lower performance on quality measures and higher mortality for CHF (30-day mortality 13.4% vs 10.9%, OR 1.28 [CI 95% 1.23–1.32]). Limited access to health care centers, absence of physicians, and lack of frequent outpatient monitoring are detrimental for the quality of care in rural settings, emphasizing the need to attract and retain qualified personnel to rural health clinics.[26]

Health Care Providers' Adherence to Guidelines in the Rural Setting

The adherence of health care providers to guideline recommendations varies widely among the published data. Balieiro and colleagues[19] reported an adequate use of angiotensin-converting enzyme inhibitors (ACEi) or angiotensin II receptor blockers (ARB) in rural Brazil. However, only 62% of the patients received beta-blockers; barely 22% of patients with CHF in atrial fibrillation were receiving oral anticoagulation.

These results contrast with those reported by Jordan and colleagues[27] in rural Australian women. This paper compared medical management of 944 women aged 77 to 83 years with self-reported CHF, ischemic cardiomyopathy, or atrial fibrillation with those recommended by clinical guidelines. For those with CHF, only 32% were receiving ACEi. Women from rural communities had higher odds of reporting never having seen a cardiologist (OR 3.88, 95% CI 1.72–8.72) and never having had an echocardiogram (OR 2.86, 95% CI 1.42–5.75) when compared with urban women. Underuse of recommended therapy by rural health care providers has also been reported in Canada[28] and Germany.[29] Therapeutic adherence seems to be low in both rural and urban patients. In a large Canadian cohort of 10,430 patients, rural patients were less likely to be adherent to ACEi/ARB, although the differences were small.[30] The implementation of nationwide policies to ensure guideline-recommended therapy is likely to have a positive effect on improving CHF quality of care as has been observed for CAD with the Get with the Guidelines-CAD Program.[31]

Organizational issues are also critical to ensure proper quality of care in CHF. In a small study of 23 US rural hospitals, higher nurse turnover was related to lower compliance with discharge instructions, lower rates of smoking cessation, and a lower rate of prescribing ACEi on discharge.[32]

Even when there is consistent evidence of impaired pharmacotherapy in the rural setting,[7] this finding alone does not explain the adverse outcomes observed in rural patients with CHF.[15] Patient-related factors, such as slowness to adopt healthy behaviors[33] and lower levels of health literacy,[34] as well as organizational factors (decreased physician density, increased propensity to use acute care facilities in rural communities[35]) contribute to increasing the number of major adverse cardiovascular events after CHF discharge in a rural setting.

PATIENT-RELATED FACTORS IN RURAL COMMUNITIES

Lack of expedited access to health care in rural areas puts further stress on the importance of self-care. Even when knowledge about the disease is insufficient by itself to ensure proper therapeutic adherence, it is the minimal requirement to promote behavioral changes associated with self-care.[36] Dracup and colleagues[37] investigated the level of knowledge about CHF in 612 patients from rural communities in California. Older men scored significantly lower, with the most frequent incorrect items related to symptoms of CHF and the need for daily weights, both critical elements to identify early decompensation and avoid preventable hospitalizations. Similarly, Moser and

colleagues[34] evaluated 575 rural patients hospitalized for heart failure within the last 6 months. In this cohort, inadequate health literacy was associated with an increase in 1.91 times the risk for rehospitalization caused by CHF or all-cause death, even after adjustment for depression, comorbidities, or worse functional class.

ROLE OF INTERVENTIONS TO IMPROVE CHRONIC HEART FAILURE OUTCOMES IN RURAL COMMUNITIES
Simplified Diagnostic Approach

The combination of reduced resource availability, lack of trained nurses and physicians and low awareness for CHF among health care providers and general population has motivated the elaboration of simplified diagnostic algorithms suitable for large-scale screening. Even when echocardiography remains the standard technique for detection of abnormal cardiac function in subjects complaining for dyspnea, its availability in rural settings is significantly lower, even in developed countries.[27] Trained nurses applying a simplified echocardiographic assessment may increase CHF diagnosis in underserved rural areas in countries in development.[38] In low- and middle-income countries, particularly in rural communities, the use of natriuretic peptides can be used both as a surrogate criterion for CHF diagnosis as well as an indication to initiate empirical CHF therapy where echocardiography is unavailable.[39] This approach has been validated by the Screening To Prevent Heart Failure Study (STOP-HF[40]) and the NT-proBNP selected prevention of cardiac events in a population of diabetic patients without a history of cardiac disease (PONTIAC)[41] trials, which showed that increased natriuretic peptide levels are associated with increased cardiovascular events and increased prevalence of CHF, even in subjects with normal echocardiograms. The use of ACEi and beta-blockers commonly used in CHF treatment reduced significantly the rate of major cardiovascular events.

Telemedicine Support

Assuring an appropriate standard of care for rural patients implies the recruitment of trained care providers, availability of diagnostic and therapeutic resources, and adequate outpatient and home-based care. Considering the evidence that hospitals within a hospital system relate to improved clinical outcomes,[42] a policy promoting partnership between rural providers and tertiary care centers is likely to have a positive effect on CHF care.[43]

Within the strategies to provide an effective partnership, telemedicine seems to be a feasible tool to improve CHF quality of care in rural settings, facilitating the delivery of health services as well as the delivery of education and teaching programs to rural health care providers.[44] A Cochrane review concluded that telemonitoring can reduce CHF-related hospitalizations and, to a more modest extent, all-cause hospitalizations.[45] However, large studies, such as the Telemonitoring in Heart Failure[46] and Telemedical Interventional Modeling in Heart Failure, have failed to demonstrate a positive effect on mortality or hospitalizations, raising considerable doubts about the real usefulness of telemedicine in CHF.[47]

However, there is considerable heterogeneity in telemedicine implementation in terms of staff, equipment, telecommunications, technical support, and training[44] that can explain the considerable dispersion of reported results. In the United States, the implementation of a telemedicine program (Care Beyond Walls and Wires) in an underserved rural area was associated with a reduction in health care utilization but without significant differences with a matched cohort.[48] In Germany, community medicine nurses train their patients to use telecare devices, such as one-lead electrocardiogram, electric scale, and tonometry, which has positively impacted general practice by actively decreasing the workload of frequent home visits in rural areas.[49]

The Chronic Heart Failure Assistance by Telephone study (CHAT) evaluated a nurse-led telephone-monitoring CHF management strategy. Although the trial failed to show differences in the Packer composite score, the telephone-monitoring program reduced the number of hospitalizations in rural patients with CHF. The CHAT trial also accounted for an often neglected aspect in telemonitoring, namely, the acceptance of the target population to remote monitoring. In this trial, only 3% of the elderly subjects were unable to learn or use the technology; overall, telemonitoring received a high acceptability rate and good adherence for least 12 months.[50] Australian guidelines recommend nurse-led, multidisciplinary CHF programs as a critical element of the standard of care in CHF. Even when ideally all patients would be exposed to at least one face-to-face home visit, the need to provide appropriate care in remote areas offers opportunity for telemonitoring to reduce the gap in rural health care.[51]

Patient Education

Lack of CHF knowledge has been identified as a major predictor for rehospitalization. Rural patients with CHF exhibit poor self-care, low levels of health literacy, and limited health care access; therefore, the potential impact of a multidisciplinary approach

to promote self-care behaviors may be more important the in urban settings.[52] A small trial with a simplified educational intervention in the United States showed that knowledge and self-care behavior related to daily weights improved significantly at 3 months in the rural patients with CHF.[53] In Japan, a multidisciplinary in-hospital CHF management program reduced in nearly 75% the incidence of a composite endpoint of hospitalization and all-cause mortality in rural CHF patients (adjusted HR 0.272, 95% CI 0.130–0.570, $P<.01$).[54] Two ongoing trials will evaluate the impact of educational programs in rural patients with CHF in the United States[55] and Thailand.[56]

Even when most studies suggest that education favorably impacts CHF outcomes, the larger Coordinating Study Evaluating Outcomes of Advising and Counseling in Heart Failure (COACH) study[57] failed to demonstrate that disease management by a nurse specializing in management of patients with CHF reduced the combined end points of death and hospitalization because of CHF compared with standard follow-up. However, patients included in the COACH trial were already in optimal therapy compared with usual care in rural settings, which may explain the larger effect observed in rural communities.

Primary Health Care Provider Education and Training

The impact of education to rural health providers on CHF outcomes is more controversial. In Spain, a structured educational course showed a positive impact of education on quality of medical history, clinical examination, laboratory tests, and treatment.[58] These results contrast with those reported by a randomized controlled trial of a quality-improvement educational program involving 47 rural hospitals in Texas that showed no incremental benefit in quality of care after the implementation of Web-based benchmarking and case-review tools.[59] Factors potentially associated with this negative result are incomplete participation of the health care staff in the educational program and high staff turnover, which is particularly evident in rural settings.[60]

SUMMARY

Patients with CHF living in rural areas face an increased risk of adverse cardiovascular events. Even in countries with universal access to health care, rural areas are characteristically underserved, with reduced health care providers supply, greater distance to health care centers, decreased physician density with higher reliance on generalists, and high health care staff turnover. On the other hand, patient-related characteristics, such as socioeconomic status, educational characteristics, and health literacy, vary widely among published data, which may explain the heterogeneity in the literature regarding rural health care. The challenge to improve rural CHF management involves multidisciplinary support to optimize CHF diagnosis, use of new monitoring technologies, improved therapeutic guideline adherence, and optimized outpatient self-management to reduce hospitalizations and death and improve the quality of life of rural patients with CHF.

REFERENCES

1. Yusuf S, Reddy S, Ounpuu S, et al. Global burden of cardiovascular diseases: part I: general considerations, the epidemiologic transition, risk factors, and impact of urbanization. Circulation 2001; 104(22):2746–53.
2. Gibson MA, Gurmu E. Rural to urban migration is an unforeseen impact of development intervention in ethiopia. PLoS One 2012;7(11):e48708.
3. Yusuf S, Rangarajan S, Teo K, et al. Cardiovascular risk and events in 17 low-, middle-, and high-income countries. N Engl J Med 2014;371(9):818–27.
4. Weeks WB, Kazis LE, Shen Y, et al. Differences in health-related quality of life in rural and urban veterans. Am J Public Health 2004;94(10):1762–7.
5. Chan L, Hart LG, Goodman DC. Geographic access to health care for rural Medicare beneficiaries. J Rural Health 2006;22(2):140–6.
6. Gibson TC, White KL, Klainer LM. The prevalence of congestive heart failure in two rural communities. J Chronic Dis 1966;19(2):141–52.
7. Clark RA, Eckert KA, Stewart S, et al. Rural and urban differentials in primary care management of chronic heart failure: new data from the CASE study. Med J Aust 2007;186(9):441–5.
8. Yang YN, Ma YT, Liu F. Incidence and distributing feature of chronic heart failure in adult population of Xinjiang. Zhonghua Xin Xue Guan Bing Za Zhi 2010;38(5):460–4 [in Chinese].
9. Méndez GF, Cowie MR. The epidemiological features of heart failure in developing countries: a review of the literature. Int J Cardiol 2001;80(2–3):213–9.
10. Bocchi EA, Arias A, Verdejo H, et al. The reality of heart failure in Latin America. J Am Coll Cardiol 2013;62(11):949–58.
11. Torio CM, Andrews RM. Geographic variation in potentially preventable hospitalizations for acute and chronic conditions, 2005–2011: statistical brief #178. Rockville (MD): Agency for Health Care Policy and Research (US); 2006.
12. Wu J-R, Moser DK, Rayens MK, et al. Rurality and event-free survival in patients with heart failure. Heart Lung 2010;39(6):512–20.
13. Harris DE, Aboueissa A-M, Hartley D. Myocardial infarction and heart failure hospitalization rates in Maine, USA - variability along the urban-rural continuum. Rural Remote Health 2008;8(2):980.
14. Teng T-HK, Katzenellenbogen JM, Hung J, et al. Rural-urban differentials in 30-day and 1-year mortality following first-ever heart failure hospitalisation in Western Australia: a population-based study using data linkage. BMJ Open 2014;4(5):e004724.
15. Gamble JM, Eurich DT, Ezekowitz JA, et al. Patterns of care and outcomes differ for urban versus rural patients with newly diagnosed heart failure, even in a universal healthcare system. Circ Heart Fail 2011;4(3):317–23.
16. Nesbitt T, Doctorvaladan S, Southard JA, et al. Correlates of quality of life in rural patients with heart failure. Circ Heart Fail 2014;7(6):882–7.
17. Ariely R, Evans K, Mills T. Heart failure in China: a review of the literature. Drugs 2013;73(7):689–701.
18. Castro P, Verdejo H, Garces E, et al. Influence of social and cultural factors in the late course of patients with congestive heart failure. Rev Chil Cardiol 2009; 28(1):51–62.
19. Balieiro HM, Osuque RK, Rangel SP, et al. Clinical and demographic profile and quality indicators for heart failure in a rural area. Arq Bras Cardiol 2009; 93(6):637–42, 687–91.
20. Page K, Lee R, Grenfell R, et al. A systematic approach to chronic heart failure care: a consensus statement. Med J Aust 2014;201(3):146–50.
21. Burgdorf F, Sundmacher L. Potentially avoidable hospital admissions in Germany: an analysis of factors influencing rates of ambulatory care sensitive hospitalizations. Dtsch Arztebl Int 2014;111(13):215–23.
22. Rabinowitz HK, Diamond JJ, Markham FW, et al. Critical factors for designing programs to increase the supply and retention of rural primary care physicians. JAMA 2001;286(9):1041–8.
23. Hernandez AF, Greiner MA, Fonarow GC, et al. Relationship between early physician follow-up and 30-day readmission among Medicare beneficiaries hospitalized for heart failure. JAMA 2010;303(17): 1716–22.
24. Muus KJ, Knudson A, Klug MG, et al. Effect of post-discharge follow-up care on re-admissions among US veterans with congestive heart failure: a rural-urban comparison. Rural Remote Health 2010; 10(2):1447.
25. Kociol RD, Greiner MA, Fonarow GC, et al. Associations of patient demographic characteristics and regional physician density with early physician follow-up among Medicare beneficiaries hospitalized with heart failure. Am J Cardiol 2011;108(7):985–91.
26. Agiro A, Wan TTH, Ortiz J. Organizational and environmental correlates to preventive quality of care in US rural health clinics. J Prim Care Community Health 2012;3(4):264–71.

27. Jordan S, Wilson A, Dobson A. Management of heart conditions in older rural and urban Australian women. Intern Med J 2011;41(10):722–9.

28. Sanborn MD, Manuel DG, Ciechanska E, et al. Potential gaps in congestive heart failure management in a rural hospital. Can J Rural Med 2005;10(3):155–61.

29. Taubert G, Bergmeier C, Andresen H, et al. Clinical profile and management of heart failure: rural community hospital vs. metropolitan heart center. Eur J Heart Fail 2001;3(5):611–7.

30. Murphy GK, McAlister FA, Eurich DT. Cardiovascular medication utilization and adherence among heart failure patients in rural and urban areas: a retrospective cohort study. Can J Cardiol 2015;31(3):341–7.

31. Ambardekar AV, Fonarow GC, Dai D, et al. Quality of care and in-hospital outcomes in patients with coronary heart disease in rural and urban hospitals (from Get With the Guidelines–Coronary Artery Disease Program). Am J Cardiol 2010;105(2):139–43.

32. Newhouse RP, Dennison Himmelfarb C, Morlock L, et al. A phased cluster-randomized trial of rural hospitals testing a quality collaborative to improve heart failure care: organizational context matters. Med Care 2013;51(5):396–403.

33. Pearson TA, Lewis C. Rural epidemiology: insights from a rural population laboratory. Am J Epidemiol 1998;148(10):949–57.

34. Moser DK, Robinson S, Biddle MJ, et al. Health literacy predicts morbidity and mortality in rural patients with heart failure. J Card Fail 2015;1–26. http://dx.doi.org/10.1016/j.cardfail.2015.04.004.

35. Jin Y, Quan H, Cujec B, et al. Rural and urban outcomes after hospitalization for congestive heart failure in Alberta, Canada. J Card Fail 2003;9(4):278–85.

36. Lainscak M, Blue L, Clark AL, et al. Self-care management of heart failure: practical recommendations from the Patient Care Committee of the Heart Failure Association of the European Society of Cardiology. Eur Heart J 2014;13(2):115–26.

37. Dracup K, Moser DK, Pelter MM, et al. Rural patients' knowledge about heart failure. J Cardiovasc Nurs 2014;29(5):423–8.

38. Kwan GF, Bukhman AK, Miller AC, et al. A simplified echocardiographic strategy for heart failure diagnosis and management within an integrated non-communicable disease clinic at district hospital level for sub-Saharan Africa. JACC Heart Fail 2013;1(3):230–6.

39. Glezeva N, Gallagher J, Ledwidge M, et al. Heart failure in sub-Saharan Africa: review of the aetiology of heart failure and the role of point-of-care biomarker diagnostics. Trop Med Int Health 2015; 20(5):581–8.

40. Ledwidge M, Gallagher J, Conlon C, et al. Natriuretic peptide–based screening and collaborative care for heart failure: the STOP-HF randomized trial. JAMA 2013;310(1):66–74.

41. Huelsmann M, Neuhold S, Resl M, et al. PONTIAC (NT-proBNP selected prevention of cardiac events in a population of diabetic patients without a history of cardiac disease). J Am Coll Cardiol 2013;62(15):1365–72.

42. Chukmaitov AS, Bazzoli GJ, Harless DW, et al. Variations in inpatient mortality among hospitals in different system types, 1995 to 2000. Med Care 2009;47(4):466–73.

43. Joynt KE, Harris Y, Orav EJ, et al. Quality of care and patient outcomes in critical access rural hospitals. JAMA 2011;306(1):1–17.

44. Smith AC, Bensink M, Armfield N, et al. Telemedicine and rural health care applications. J Postgrad Med 2005;51(4):286.

45. Inglis SC, Clark RA, McAlister FA, et al. Which components of heart failure programmes are effective? A systematic review and meta-analysis of the outcomes of structured telephone support or tele-monitoring as the primary component of chronic heart failure management in 8323 patients: abridged Cochrane Review. Eur J Heart Fail 2011;13(9):1028–40.

46. Chaudhry SI, Mattera JA, Curtis JP, et al. Telemonitoring in patients with heart failure. N Engl J Med 2010;363(24):2301–9.

47. Dierckx R, Pellicori P, Cleland JGF, et al. Telemonitoring in heart failure: big brother watching over you. Heart Fail Rev 2015;20(1):107–16.

48. Riley WT, Keberlein P, Sorenson G, et al. Program evaluation of remote heart failure monitoring: healthcare utilization analysis in a rural regional medical center. Telemed J E Health 2015;21(3):157–62.

49. Terschüren C, Fendrich K, van den Berg N, et al. Implementing telemonitoring in the daily routine of a GP practice in a rural setting in northern Germany. J Telemed Telecare 2007;13(4):197–201.

50. Krum H, Forbes A, Yallop J, et al. Telephone support to rural and remote patients with heart failure: the Chronic Heart Failure Assessment by Telephone (CHAT) study. Cardiovasc Ther 2013;31(4):230–7.

51. Stewart S. Nurse-led care of heart failure: will it work in remote settings? Heart Lung Circ 2012;21(10):644–7.

52. McAlister FA, Stewart S, Ferrua S, et al. Multidisciplinary strategies for the management of heart failure patients at high risk for admission: a systematic review of randomized trials. J Am Coll Cardiol 2004;44(4):810–9.

53. Caldwell MA, Peters KJ, Dracup KA. A simplified education program improves knowledge, self-care behavior, and disease severity in heart failure patients in rural settings. Am Heart J 2005;150(5):983.e7–12.

54. Kinugasa Y, Kato M, Sugihara S, et al. Multidisciplinary intensive education in the hospital improves outcomes for hospitalized heart failure patients in a

Japanese rural setting. BMC Health Serv Res 2014; 14(1):351–9.

55. Young L, Barnason S, Do V. Promoting self-management through adherence among heart failure patients discharged from rural hospitals: a study protocol. F1000Res 2014;1–12. http://dx.doi.org/10.12688/f1000research.5998.1.

56. Srisuk N, Cameron J, Ski CF, et al. Trial of a family-based education program for heart failure patients in rural Thailand. BMC Cardiovasc Disord 2014; 14(1):173–9.

57. Jaarsma T, van der Wal MHL, Lesman-Leegte I, et al. Effect of moderate or intensive disease management program on outcome in patients with heart failure: Coordinating Study Evaluating Outcomes of Advising and Counseling in Heart Failure (COACH). Arch Intern Med 2008;168(3):316–24.

58. Velasco J, Nielsen AM. Quality of care of patients with chronic heart failure in primary care. Semergen 2012;38(3):151–9 [in Spanish].

59. Filardo G, Nicewander D, Herrin J, et al. A hospital-randomized controlled trial of a formal quality improvement educational program in rural and small community Texas hospitals: one year results. Int J Qual Health Care 2009;21(4):225–32.

60. Filardo G, Nicewander D, Herrin J, et al. Challenges in conducting a hospital-randomized trial of an educational quality improvement intervention in rural and small community hospitals. Am J Med Qual 2008;23(6):440–7.

Inequalities in the Access to Advanced Therapy in Heart Failure

Douglas Greig, MD, MSc*, Gabriel Olivares, MD

KEYWORDS

- Advanced heart failure • Implantable cardioverter-defibrillator • Cardiac resynchronization therapy
- Heart transplant • Mechanical cardiac support

KEY POINTS

- Advanced heart failure is the final stage of the disease and its recognition is clinically relevant because its short survival and limited therapies.
- Currently, heart transplantation remains as the gold standard treatment of advanced heart failure patients; however, other therapies (i.e. Mechanical cardiac support, access to specialist care) are widely available in developed countries.
- In developing countries there are several difficulties in the access to more advances therapies. Some of them are related to the relatively low budget expended on health, and other are related to health policies and academic issues.

INTRODUCTION

At present, heart failure (HF) is a worldwide problem, characterized by a high morbidity and mortality. In industrialized countries or regions, such as the United States, Canada, and western European countries, HF has a prevalence of 1.5% to 2.7% and represents the first cause of hospitalization in patients older than 65 years.[1] Moreover, according to US forecasting analyses, the total cost of care for HF will increase 3-fold by 2030.[2] On the other hand, in Chile—a middle-income country with a population estimated at 17.63 millions—the prevalence of HF is estimated at 3% and is responsible for almost 12,500 hospital discharges, accounting for 38% of the cardiovascular discharges in the country.[3]

Chile represents a growing economy in Latin America; however, the relatively high cost of more advanced therapies, in addition to other variables (ie, adequate and timely evaluation by HF specialists), makes access difficult for patients with HF. In this article, the authors review the principal difficulties in accessing advanced HF therapies in Chile, as a model of developing country.

SOME DEFINITIONS
Developing Countries

The World Bank classifies world's economies based on estimates of gross national incomes (GNIs). According to this organization, Chile has recently become a high-income country (with a GNI per capita > US $12,616). However, there is no single definition for these concepts.[4] For example, the International Monetary Fund (IMF) classifies Chile as a developing economy based on several parameters (ie, per capita income, exports diversification, and integration in the global market). According to the IMF, in 2014, the gross domestic product (GDP) per capita was Int$22,971 compared with Int$54,597 in the

The authors have nothing to disclose.
Division of Cardiovascular Diseases, P Universidad Católica de Chile, Hospital Clínico UC, 367 Marcoleta St. 8th floor, Santiago 8330024, Chile
* Corresponding author. Hospital Clínico UC, Marcoleta 367, 8th Floor, Santiago 8330024, Chile.
E-mail address: dgreig@puc.cl

Heart Failure Clin 11 (2015) 523–528
http://dx.doi.org/10.1016/j.hfc.2015.07.014

United States and Int$44,854 in Canada. Moreover, Chilean health costs represent 7.7% of the GDP compared with 17.7% in the United States and 10.9% in Canada.[5] On the other hand, the United Nations (UN) Human Development Index (HDI)—involving income, life expectancy, and education—classifies Chile as a very high human developed country (eg, HDI estimate in 2013 was 0.822 in Chile, compared with 0.914 in the United States). In 2013, this UN program reported a life expectancy in Chile of 80 years compared with 78.9 years in the United States and 81.5 years in Canada.[6,7]

The Chilean Health Care Model, as a Model of a Developing Country

In Chile there is a dual coverage system. The National Health Care Fund covered 69% of the population in 2013 and is administrated by the government. Also, in 2012, 49% of health spending was funded by public source, far below the average of 72% in the Organization for Economic Cooperation and Development (OECD). On the other hand, private health insurance companies covered 17% of the population. Unfortunately, this dual health system (public and private) which encourages that high-risk and lower-income patients are covered by the government; however, its relatively low budget prevents access to more expensive therapies.[8] Moreover, in 2004, the Chilean government introduced a medical benefit package in which almost 80 diseases are covered with a minimum of treatments; HF, however, was not included.[9]

Defining Advanced Heart Failure

A concise definition of advanced HF is difficult because its progression is highly variable and the exact course is uncertain.[10] According to the Heart Failure Society of America, advanced HF (or stage D) can be defined "as the presence of progressive and/or persistent severe signs and symptoms of HF despite optimized medical, surgical and device therapy. It is generally accompanied by frequent hospitalization, severely limited exercise tolerance, poor quality of life and high morbid-mortality."[11] Advanced HF usually involves heart structural abnormalities and rest symptoms, and frequently requires advanced therapies, such as continuous infusion of inotropes or diuretics (even when the patient is at home), mechanical cardiac support, heart transplant (HTx), and experimental therapies. Therefore, identification of these patients is clinically and prognostically relevant to promptly initiate adequate therapeutic strategies.[12] Although several biomarkers, hemodynamic data,

and prognostic models have been used in an attempt to identify the transition to advanced HF, none have proven to be useful in the clinical setting. Examples of prognostic factors include demographics (eg, age, sex), functional class, exercise capacity (ie, peak oxygen consumption), left ventricular ejection fraction, filling pressures, results of renal and liver dysfunction tests, and levels of biomarkers (eg, inflammatory, pro-brain natriuretic peptide), among others. Even though more sophisticated prognostic models (eg, Heart Failure Survival Score, Seattle Heart Failure Survival Score, Enhanced Feedback for Effective Cardiac Treatment (EFFECT) Heart Failure Mortality Prediction) have been proved to provide more refined predictions of prognosis in hospitalized and ambulatory patients with HF, there is no clear consensus on what is the expected survival that defines advanced HF.[12–16] In addition, there are no good data regarding prevalence.[17] The cohort from Olmstead County shows that only 0.2% of patients with HF were in stage D.[18] The quality of life and the prognosis are poor. In addition, once patients reach stage D, mortality ranges from 79% to 89% in 1 year.[19]

GENERAL APPROACH TO ADVANCED THERAPIES AND INTRODUCTION TO THE PROBLEM OF INEQUALITIES

Characteristics that guarantee a more aggressive approach in patients with advanced HF are worsening symptoms, frequent hospitalizations, and intolerance to up titration of medications, among others. However, there is no single event that suggests a transition to advanced HF. Over the past decade, different scientific societies and guidelines have proposed some patterns of clinical characteristics that suggest that patients are getting worse (ie, failure of optimal and surgical therapy) and should be referred for more advanced evaluations and therapies (**Box 1**). At this stage, all the patients should be on optimal and evidence-based therapies.[11,20]

Cardiac Resynchronization Therapy and Implantable Cardioverter-Defibrillators

In HF, almost half of the deaths are attributable to ventricular arrhythmias. Several trials have demonstrated that prophylactic implantation of an implantable cardioverter-defibrillator (ICD) can decrease the mortality in about 10%.[21,22] However, some trials suggest that such benefit is not seen in patients with more advanced HF, and there is no demonstrated improvement in symptoms or quality of life.[11] For these reasons, current guidelines do not support the indication of an ICD if the patient's

---

Box 1
Indicators of advanced HF (triggers)

- Need for intravenous inotropic therapy for symptomatic relief or to maintain end-organ function
- Peak Vo_2 less than 14 mL/kg/min or less than 50% of predicted
- The 6-min walk distance less than 300 m
- Two or more HF admissions in 12 months
- More than 2 unscheduled visits (eg, ED or clinic) in 12 months
- Worsening right-sided HF and secondary pulmonary hypertension
- Diuretic refractoriness associated with worsening renal function
- Circulatory renal limitation to RAAS inhibition or β-blocker therapy
- Progressive/persistent NYHA functional class III–IV symptoms
- Increased 1-year mortality (eg, 20%–25%) predicted by HF survival models (eg, SHFM, HFSS, etc)
- Progressive renal or hepatic end-organ dysfunction
- Persistent hyponatremia (serum sodium levels <134 mEq/L)
- Recurrent refractory ventricular tachyarrhythmias; frequent ICD shocks
- Cardiac cachexia
- Inability to perform ADL

Abbreviations: ADL, activities of daily living; ED, emergency department; HFSS, Heart Failure Survival Score; ICD, implantable cardioverter-defibrillator; NYHA, New York Heart Association; RAAS, renin angiotensin aldosterone system; SFHM, Seattle Heart Failure Survival Score; Vo_2, oxygen consumption.
 Data from Stewart GC, Givertz MM. Mechanical circulatory support for advanced heart failure: patients and technology in evolution. Circulation 2012;125(10):1304–15; and Fang JC, Ewald GA, Allen LA, et al. Advanced (stage d) heart failure: a statement from the heart failure society of America guidelines committee. J Card Fail 2015;21(6):519–34.

---

life expectancy is less than 1 year.[23] Conversely, in a subset of patients with advanced HF enrolled in the Comparison of Medical Therapy, Pacing, and Defibrillation in Heart Failure (COMPANION) trial, cardiac resynchronization therapy (CRT) and CRT plus defibrillation (CRT-D) therapy shows a trend for improvement in survival and delayed time for hospitalization.[24] Similarly, Hansky and colleagues[25] show—in patients with HF who are candidates for HTx—that CRT can extend the waiting period without effect on the overall survival. The relatively high initial payments are usually not covered by health programs in Latin America, therefore the indications should be restricted to patients who will obtain more benefits. For example, a Brazilian study found that ICD becomes cost effective in highly selected patients, than in those with more wide indication criteria (incremental cost-effectiveness ratio [ICER] of Int$18,000 per quality-adjusted life-year [QALY] gained compared with > Int$50,000 per QALY gained, respectively). A similar situation has been observed in CRT implantations.[26] Therefore, both ICD and CRT-D could be cost effective in Chile and other Latin America countries based on a strict strategy in the selection of patients.

Mechanical Cardiac Support

At present, short-term devices are widely available and usually covered in the authors' country. However, the availability of more durable ventricular assist devices (VADs) is still limited. At present, VADs are indicated mainly as bridge-to-transplant (BTT) devices or as permanent devices (destination therapy). The actuarial survival of patient with continuous flow pumps is 80% at 1 year and 70% at 2 years.[27] According to VAD manufacturers, there have now been more than 24,000 continuous flow devices implanted.[11] According to Miller and colleagues,[28] the number of candidates to receive left ventricular assist device (LVAD) in the United States may be as high as 250,000 to 300,000. Using a similar methodology, it can be estimated that there are 12,000 potential candidates of LVAD in Chile. In developed countries, it is widely accepted that a therapy with an ICER less than US $60,000 is very acceptable and one with an ICER greater than US $100,000 is unattractive.[29] Contemporary studies show that using VADs as BTT devices increases survival at increased cost relative to using nonbridged HTx. A recent study by Alba and colleagues[30] shows a cost-effectiveness ratio (CER) of canadian dollars (CAD)$84,964 per life-year in high-risk patients and CAD$119,574 per-life year in low-risk patients. To the authors' knowledge, there are no long-term cost-effectiveness studies on VADs in Latin America. However, some regional economic evaluations suggest a willingness-to-pay level around US $50,000 per QALY to be considered as an acceptable therapy.[26] Consequently, the high cost of VADs is one major factor to limit its availability in the authors' country, and the region. These data are reflected in the fact that since the first implant in 2013, no more than 10 VADs (in 4 different centers) have been installed in Chile. All VADs, except 2, have been paid as a part of exceptional funds provided by the government or donations by nonprofit institutions.

Heart Transplant

HTx remains the gold standard therapeutic option for patients with advanced HF. The median survival is 13 years for those patients who survive the first year.[31] The number of transplants has remained stable since 2005, and most centers (77%) perform less than 20 HTxs per year.[32] The information regarding effective donor rates in Latin America is scarce. Data from 2004 report an effective deceased organ donor rate in Latin America of 5.4 per million.[33] Conversely, in Canada, in 2014, there were 15.5 deceased organ donors per million population, an increase of 17% since 2003.[34]

In Chile, the donation rate has decreased since 2006 (from 10 deceased organ donors per million population to 7 in 2014, **Fig. 1**), causing an increase of the HTx waiting list time.[35] This increase in turn has resulted in an increased number of patients on the waiting list. In Chile, HTx is well covered by the public and private health system. The situation is similar in most Latin American countries. However, there is a great variability in the treatments included, particularly in the follow-up.[26] In the authors' opinion, in Chile, HTx continues to be the gold standard treatment of advanced HF with excellent survival and functional status results.[36,37]

OTHER FACTORS THAT MAKE DIFFICULT THE ACCESS TO ADVANCED THERAPIES
Economic Issues

Over the past 10 years, the budget expended on health has increased from 6.7% in 2005 to 7.7% of GDP in 2013. This expenditure is slightly higher than that of similar countries in Latin America (eg, Argentina health expenditure was 7.3% of GDP in 2013) but still lower than those of other more developed countries in the region (eg, Brazil health expenditure was 9.7% of GDP in 2013) or other developed countries (eg, the US and Canada health expenditures were 17.1% and 11.1% of GDP in 2013, respectively).[38] On the other hand, national programs focus on stages A and B of HF. For example, arterial hypertension, coronary disease, and diabetes mellitus are covered by GES in both public and private health systems. However, once advanced symptoms are developed, there are no plans that specifically cover these patients. More concerning is the situation of terminal patients, where the plans are only focused on patients with advanced cancer.[9]

Access to Health Care

In terms of HF programs in clinics, there are only 2 public programs for the whole country. One of them is a reference center serving a population of 17 million. The situation is not different in the private health system where, to the authors' knowledge, there are not specific heart function programs. On the other hand, Chile has 6 private and 2 public centers that perform HTxs. All, except one, are located in Santiago (capital of Chile). In contrast, in countries with 100% public-covered systems, there is an increased access to health

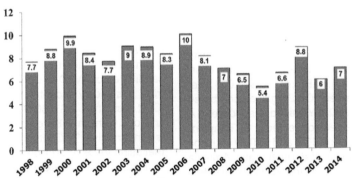

Fig. 1. Trend in the deceased organ donors in Chile (1998–2014). Annual rate per million population.

care—including HF programs—for a substantial proportion of the population.[26,39] By September 2014, the Chilean Ministry of Health reported a waiting list for cardiology of 52,355 patients (representing 3.4% of the total waiting list in the country). Of them, 74% of the patients have been waiting for more than 120 days.[40] The lack of specialized centers both in sufficient and widely available number, and the long waiting lists, make access to reasonable advanced therapies difficult.

Low Number of Heart Failure Specialists

According to OECD Health Statistics, the supply of health workers in Chile is low compared with that in developed countries. In 2012, there were 1.7 doctors per 1000 population, compared with 2.5 per 1000 in Canada and the United States. Moreover, a recent study shows that only 2.1% (n = 789) of the specialists are registered cardiologists.[8] Moreover, the National Board of Medical Specialties does not recognize specialization in HF or cardiac transplant. Consequently, specialists should apply abroad in order to get an internationally recognized subspecialization. In addition, in the past decade, there were cardiology specialties program for nursing; however, these programs are oriented at the acute and intensive setting.

SUMMARY

In developing countries, particularly in Latin America, there are several difficulties in the access to more advanced therapies. The main issues at hand are economic issues, lack of appropriate and widely available programs, and the relatively low number of HF specialists (ie, making access to appropriate health care more difficult). These inequalities, compared to more developed countries, should encourage the development of academic, teaching, and cost-effectiveness programs based on the local reality. The authors think that these programs should include new long-term technology (ie, VADs) and should be financed by national health systems.

REFERENCES

1. Roger VL, Go AS, Lloyd-Jones DM, et al. Heart disease and stroke statistics–2012 update: a report from the American Heart Association. Circulation 2012;125(1):e2–220.
2. Heidenreich PA, Albert NM, Allen LA, et al. Forecasting the impact of heart failure in the United States: a policy statement from the American Heart Association. Circ Heart Fail 2013;6(3):606–19.
3. V R. Chilean Heart Failure Guidelines. 2015. Available at: http://wwwsochicarcl/indexphp/educacioncontinua-mainmenu-51/gu-de-manejo-clco-mainmenu-60/insuficiencia-carda-y-transplante-mainmenu-233html. Accessed July, 2015.
4. DATA WB. GNI per capita, PPP. 2015. Available at: http://data.worldbank.org/indicator/NY.GNP.PCAP.PP.CD. Accessed July, 2015.
5. Fund IM. World economic outlook. IMF. 2015. Available at: http://www.imf.org/external/pubs/ft/weo/2015/01/pdf/text.pdf. Accessed July, 2015.
6. Program UND. Human Development Report, Sustained Human Progress. 2014. Available at: http://hdr.undp.org/sites/default/files/hdr14-report-en-1.pdf. Accessed July, 2015.
7. Program UND. Table 1. Human Development Index and its components. 2015. Available at: http://hdr.undp.org/es/content/table-1-human-development-index-and-its-components. Accessed July, 2015.
8. Economic Of, Development C-oa. OECD Health Statistics 2014 How does Chile compare? 2014. Available at: http://www.oecd.org/els/health-systems/Briefing-Note-CHILE-2014.pdf. Accessed July, 2015.
9. Ministry of Health C. Patologías garantizadas AUGE. 2015. Available at: http://www.supersalud.gob.cl/difusion/572/w3-propertyname-501.html. Accessed July, 2015.
10. Gott M, Barnes S, Parker C, et al. Dying trajectories in heart failure. Palliat Med 2007;21(2):95–9.
11. Fang JC, Ewald GA, Allen LA, et al. Advanced (stage d) heart failure: a statement from the Heart Failure Society of America Guidelines Committee. J Card Fail 2015;21(6):519–34.
12. Allen LA, Stevenson LW, Grady KL, et al. Decision making in advanced heart failure: a scientific statement from the American Heart Association. Circulation 2012;125(15):1928–52.
13. Aaronson KD, Schwartz JS, Chen TM, et al. Development and prospective validation of a clinical index to predict survival in ambulatory patients referred for cardiac transplant evaluation. Circulation 1997;95(12):2660–7.
14. Greig D, Austin PC, Zhou L, et al. Ischemic electrocardiographic abnormalities and prognosis in decompensated heart failure. Circ Heart Fail 2014;7(6):986–93.
15. Lee DS, Austin PC, Rouleau JL, et al. Predicting mortality among patients hospitalized for heart failure: derivation and validation of a clinical model. JAMA 2003;290(19):2581–7.
16. Mozaffarian D, Anker SD, Anand I, et al. Prediction of mode of death in heart failure: the Seattle Heart Failure Model. Circulation 2007;116(4):392–8.
17. Ho KK, Pinsky JL, Kannel WB, et al. The epidemiology of heart failure: the Framingham Study. J Am Coll Cardiol 1993;22(4 Suppl A):6A–13A.

18. Ammar KA, Jacobsen SJ, Mahoney DW, et al. Prevalence and prognostic significance of heart failure stages: application of the American College of Cardiology/American Heart Association heart failure staging criteria in the community. Circulation 2007; 115(12):1563–70.

19. Rogers JG, Butler J, Lansman SL, et al. Chronic mechanical circulatory support for inotrope-dependent heart failure patients who are not transplant candidates: results of the INTrEPID Trial. J Am Coll Cardiol 2007;50(8):741–7.

20. Stewart GC, Givertz MM. Mechanical circulatory support for advanced heart failure: patients and technology in evolution. Circulation 2012;125(10): 1304–15.

21. Epstein AE, DiMarco JP, Ellenbogen KA, et al. ACC/AHA/HRS 2008 Guidelines for Device-Based Therapy of Cardiac Rhythm Abnormalities: a report of the American College of Cardiology/American Heart Association Task Force on Practice Guidelines (Writing Committee to Revise the ACC/AHA/NASPE 2002 Guideline Update for Implantation of Cardiac Pacemakers and Antiarrhythmia Devices) developed in collaboration with the American Association for Thoracic Surgery and Society of Thoracic Surgeons. J Am Coll Cardiol 2008;51(21):e1–62.

22. Nanthakumar K, Epstein AE, Kay GN, et al. Prophylactic implantable cardioverter-defibrillator therapy in patients with left ventricular systolic dysfunction: a pooled analysis of 10 primary prevention trials. J Am Coll Cardiol 2004;44(11):2166–72.

23. Yancy CW, Jessup M, Bozkurt B, et al. 2013 ACCF/AHA guideline for the management of heart failure: a report of the American College of Cardiology Foundation/American Heart Association Task Force on Practice Guidelines. J Am Coll Cardiol 2013; 62(16):e147–239.

24. Lindenfeld J, Feldman AM, Saxon L, et al. Effects of cardiac resynchronization therapy with or without a defibrillator on survival and hospitalizations in patients with New York Heart Association class IV heart failure. Circulation 2007;115(2):204–12.

25. Hansky B, Vogt J, Zittermann A, et al. Cardiac resynchronization therapy: long-term alternative to cardiac transplantation? Ann Thorac Surg 2009; 87(2):432–8.

26. Paim J, Travassos C, Almeida C, et al. The Brazilian health system: history, advances, and challenges. Lancet 2011;377(9779):1778–97.

27. Kirklin JK, Naftel DC, Pagani FD, et al. Sixth INTERMACS annual report: a 10,000-patient database. J Heart Lung Transplant 2014;33(6):555–64.

28. Miller LW, Guglin M, Rogers J. Cost of ventricular assist devices: can we afford the progress? Circulation 2013;127(6):743–8.

29. Goldman L, Gordon DJ, Rifkind BM, et al. Cost and health implications of cholesterol lowering. Circulation 1992;85(5):1960–8.

30. Alba AC, Alba LF, Delgado DH, et al. Cost-effectiveness of ventricular assist device therapy as a bridge to transplantation compared with nonbridged cardiac recipients. Circulation 2013;127(24):2424–35.

31. Stehlik J, Edwards LB, Kucheryavaya AY, et al. The Registry of the International Society for Heart and Lung Transplantation: twenty-seventh official adult heart transplant report–2010. J Heart Lung Transplant 2010;29(10):1089–103.

32. Stehlik J, Edwards LB, Kucheryavaya AY, et al. The Registry of the International Society for Heart and Lung Transplantation: 29th official adult heart transplant report–2012. J Heart Lung Transplant 2012; 31(10):1052–64.

33. Mizraji R, Alvarez I, Palacios RI, et al. Organ donation in Latin America. Transplant Proc 2007;39(2): 333–5.

34. Information CIfH. Canadian Organ Replacement Register Annual Report: Treatment of End-Stage Organ Failure in Canada, 2003 to 2012. 2014. Available at: https://secure.cihi.ca/free_products/2014_CORR_Annual_Report_EN.pdf. Accessed July, 2015.

35. Ministry of Health C. Datos Donantes de Órganos Junio 2015 [data on organ donors by June 2015]. 2015. Available at: http://web.minsal.cl/introduccion_trasplantes. Accessed July, 2015.

36. Moran S, Castro P, Zalaquett R, et al. Tratamiento de la insuficiencia cardiaca avanzada mediante trasplante de corazon. [Treatment of advanced heart failure by heart transplantation]. Rev Med Chil 2001;129(1):9–17 [in Spanish].

37. Villavicencio M, Rossel V, Larrea R, et al. Experiencia clinica con 53 trasplantes cardiacos consecutivos. [Clinical experience with 53 consecutive heart transplants]. Rev Med Chil 2013;141(12):1499–505 [in Spanish].

38. Bank W. Health Expenditure, total (% of GDP). 2015. Available at: http://data.worldbank.org/indicator/SH.XPD.TOTL.ZS?page=1. Accessed July, 2015.

39. Blair JE, Huffman M, Shah SJ. Heart failure in North America. Curr Cardiol Rev 2013;9(2):128–46.

40. Ministry of Health C. Lista de Espera No GES. 2014. Available at: web.minsal.cl/sites/default/files/files/image2015-04-07-165945.pdf. Accessed July, 2015.

Gaps and Resemblances in Current Heart Failure Guidelines: A Clinical Perspective

Juan F. Bulnes, MD[a], Jorge E. Jalil, MD[b],*

KEYWORDS

- Heart failure guidelines • Gaps • Heart failure treatment

KEY POINTS

- The newly available clinical guidelines in heart failure (HF) from Europe (2012), the United States (2010 and 2013), and Canada (2015) were compared.
- The focus was on the systems for grading the evidence and classifying the recommendations, HF definitions, pharmacologic treatment, and devices used in HF.
- No large gaps were evident in the methodology for assessing evidence or in HF definitions. Pharmacologic treatments and recommendations for cardiac resynchronization therapy and implantable cardioverter-defibrillators are similar. Guideline recommendations regarding new emergent treatments are becoming available.

INTRODUCTION

To contrast the levels of evidence and classes of recommendation for several pharmacologic and device therapies advocated by the different clinical guidelines in chronic heart failure (HF), McMurray and Swedberg[1] compared the 4 major guidelines in 2006. They also discussed potential explanations for discrepancies among the different guidelines.[1] Since then, more recent clinical studies in HF have provided data to renew the current recommendations with more evidence and the major clinical guidelines have been updated accordingly. Specifically, guidelines from the European Society of Cardiology (ESC) were updated in 2012,[2] guidelines from the American Heart Association (AHA)/American College of Cardiology (ACC) were updated in 2013,[3] those from the Heart Failure Society of America (HFSA) were updated in 2010,[3] and the guidelines from the Canadian Cardiovascular Society Heart Failure (CCS) were updated from 2010 to 2015.[4–8]

This article compares these 4 new clinical guidelines in HF from a clinician perspective in order to detect relevant differences and to discuss some explanations. It focuses on 4 main aspects of these guidelines: the systems of grading the evidence and classifying the recommendations, the definitions of HF, pharmacologic treatment, and devices used in HF.

GRADING THE EVIDENCE AND CLASSIFYING THE RECOMMENDATIONS

Although the systems for grading the evidence and classifying the recommendations among the AHA/ACC, ESC, HFSA, and CCS (until 2010) are similar, they are not exactly the same, but we ignored the small differences. In contrast, since 2011, the CCS guidelines use the grading of recommendations assessment, development and evaluation (GRADE) system, which, among other features, defines strength of recommendations in terms of patient choices. At present, for the CCS guidelines, both systems are still valid, as reflected in the CCS HF Web Compendium guidelines (**Table 1**).[2–9]

[a] Division of Internal Medicine, School of Medicine, Pontificia Universidad Catolica de Chile, Marcoleta 367, Santiago 8320000, Chile; [b] Division of Cardiovascular Diseases, School of Medicine, Pontificia Universidad Catolica de Chile, Marcoleta 367, 8th Floor, Santiago 8320000, Chile
* Corresponding author.
E-mail address: jjalil@med.puc.cl

Heart Failure Clin 11 (2015) 529–541
http://dx.doi.org/10.1016/j.hfc.2015.07.013

Table 1
Grading the evidence level and class of recommendations

	AHA/ACC, ESC, HFSA, and CCS (Until 2010)			CCS (Since 2011)	
	Class	**Definition**	**Suggested Wording to Use**	**Strength**	**Definition**
Class/strength of the recommendation ~ Size of treatment effect	I	Benefit>>>risk	Is recommended	Strong	Most informed patients choose the recommended management
	IIa	Benefit>>risk	Should be considered	Weak	Patients' choices vary according to their values and preferences. Clinicians must ensure that patients' care is in keeping with their values and preferences
	IIb	Benefit ≥ risk	May be considered		
	III	No benefit/harm	Is not recommended		

	AHA/ACC, ESC, HFSA, and CCS (Until 2010)		CCS (Since 2011)	
	Level	**Definition**	**Quality**	**Definition**
Level/quality of the evidence ~ Estimate of certainty of treatment effect	A	Data derived from multiple RCTs or meta-analyses	High	Further research is unlikely to change confidence in the estimate of effect
	B	Data derived from a single RCT or nonrandomized studies	Moderate	Further research is likely to affect confidence in the estimate of effect and may change the estimate
	C	Only consensus opinion of experts, case studies, or standard of care	Low	Further research is very likely to affect confidence in the estimate of effect and is likely to change the effect
			Very low	Any estimate of effect is very uncertain

Abbreviation: RCT, randomized controlled trial.

Table 2
HF: classifications and definitions

	AHA/ACC	ESC	CCS	HFSA
Systolic dysfunction (HFrEF)	EF ≤40%	EF ≤35%	EF <40%	Reduced LVEF. Sometimes: HF with a dilated left ventricle (EF not specified)
Diastolic dysfunction (HFpEF)	EF ≥50%	EF ≥50%	EF not specified	Preserved LVEF. Sometimes: HF with a nondilated LV(EF not specified)
Intermediate categories	HFpEF, borderline: EF 41%–49% HFrEF, recovered: EF >40%	Gray area	NS	NS

Abbreviations: EF, ejection fraction; HFpEF, HF with preserved ejection fraction; HFrEF, HF with reduced ejection fraction; LVEF, LV ejection fraction; NS, not specified.

DEFINITIONS AND TYPES OF HEART FAILURE

Definitions of HF types are similar among the 4 new guidelines (**Table 2**). All recognize both systolic and diastolic dysfunction, but boundaries are different among them. Although defined ejection fraction (EF) cut points are provided by the AHA/ACC and ESC guidelines for both systolic and diastolic dysfunction, CCS provides them only for left ventricular (LV) systolic dysfunction.[2–9] No precise boundaries are mentioned in the HFSA guidelines. Note that the reduced EF cut point considered by the ESC (≤35%) is more pragmatic, because it probably better represents the population included in trials with proven benefit in terms of mortality.

A second relevant difference is the recognition of an intermediate category by both the AHA/ ACC and the ESC guidelines, which is not considered by the other 2 guidelines. Although the ESC guidelines call it a gray area, characterized by mild systolic dysfunction, the AHA/ACC notably divides it into 2 different subtypes: HF with preserved EF (HFpEF) borderline, with characteristics, treatment patterns, and outcomes that seem similar to those of patients with HF with preserved EF (HFpEF); and HFrEF recovered, a subset of patients with improved and previously reduced EF that may be clinically distinct from those with persistently preserved or reduced EF.

Considerable gaps exist between major guidelines in the inclusion of preclinical stages of HF (**Table 3**). Although the 3 North American societies include asymptomatic LV dysfunction (ALVD) as a particular category of disease,[3–9] with specific

Table 3
Asymptomatic LV dysfunction (EF <40%, unless specified)

	AHA/ACC		ESC		CCS		HFSA	
Major Guideline Recommendations	Class	Level	Class	Level	Class	Level	Class	Level
ACE Inhibitors								
After MI								
EF <40%	I	A	NS	NS	I	A	I	A
Irrespective of previous MI								
EF <40%	I	A	NS	NS	NS	NS	I	A
EF <35%	NS	NS	NS	NS	Strong	MQ	NS	NS
ARB if ACE inhibitors not tolerated	I	A	NS	NS	Strong	MQ	I	C
β-Blockers								
After MI	I	B	NS	NS	I	B	IIa	B
Irrespective of previous MI	I	C	NS	NS	IIa	C	IIa	C

Abbreviations: ACE, angiotensin I–converting enzyme; ARB, angiotensin receptor blockers; MI, myocardial infarction; MQ, middle quality; NS, not specified.

Table 4
Clinical use of diuretics in HF

Major Guideline Recommendations	AHA/ACC		ESC		CCS		HFSA	
	Class	Level	Class	Level	Class	Level	Class	Level
For evidence of fluid retention: to improve symptoms, achieve and maintain euvolemia, using the lowest achievable dose	I	C	NS	NS	Strong	LQ	I	B
Loop diuretics as first-line choice	NS	NS	NS	NS	Strong	LQ	I	B
Cautious addition of thiazides or metolazone in patients with persistent fluid retention	NS	NS	NS	NS	Weak	MQ	IIa	C

Abbreviation: LQ, low quality.

recommendations (notably the 4-stage spectrum of HF proposed by the AHA/ACC guidelines), the ESC only considers symptomatic HF in its guidelines.[2]

Among the North American societies, some differences exist on recommendations for ALVD, according to its origin (ischemic [ie, after myocardial infarction (MI)] or nonischemic) and severity of LV dysfunction. For example, although the 3 societies give a class I level A recommendation for the use of angiotensin-converting enzyme (ACE) inhibitors in ALVD of ischemic origin, the CCS gives just a moderate quality recommendation for its use in nonischemic ALVD, and demands a lower EF (<35%). Fewer differences exist between the guidelines regarding the use β-blockers in this category in this clinical setting (for the key studies see Refs.[10–14]).

PHARMACOLOGIC TREATMENT IN HEART FAILURE

All 4 guidelines agree on almost every aspect regarding diuretic use (**Table 4**); however, although some of them make specific recommendations, others do not. For example, the ESC guidelines do not make any recommendation about diuretic use, although they include a section that contains the same concepts presented as specific recommendations by the other societies. Note that only the CCS supports its recommendations with evidence[1] (for key studies see Refs.[15,16]).

Angiotensin I–Converting Enzyme Inhibitors

ACE inhibitors are probably the most well-established and least controversial topic in HFrEF treatment. Agreement about recommendations for such drugs is strong among the HF guidelines

(**Table 5**). Different statements on recommendations are provided here to show that, although subtle differences in redaction do exist, they all include the same key aspects: symptomatic HF (current or prior symptoms), reduced EF, morbidity and mortality reduction, and concomitance with β-blocker use (see **Table 5**). Key studies include CONSENSUS (1987),[17] SOLVD-Treatment (1991),[18] and ATLAS (1999).[19]

Angiotensin Receptor Blockers

The 4 main indications for angiotensin receptor blockers (ARBs) in HF are shown in **Table 6**. All 4 societies agree on the use of ARBs in patients intolerant of ACE inhibitors (because of cough or angioedema, but not because of hyperkalemia or worsening renal function). More gaps exist in other areas. Only the US societies recommend use of ARBs as a reasonable, first-line alternative to ACE inhibitors, both with level of evidence A. However, within the evidence cited for this recommendation in the AHA/ACC guidelines, there is only 1 randomized controlled trial (RCT) (RESOLVD), in which mortality was not measured.[20]

In patients with HF with persistent symptoms despite ACE inhibitors and β-blockers, in view of the results of the Val-HeFT[21] and CHARM-Added[22] trials, ARBs are recommended in the HFSA guidelines as the third drug. However, the pooled evidence provided by 3 trials, EMPHASIS-HF[23] (published 1 year after HFSA guidelines), Ephesus,[24] and RALES,[25] favor mineralocorticoid receptor antagonists (MRA) as the third drug of choice. Thus, the AHA, ESC, and CCS guidelines consider ARB as the third drug of choice in the setting of patients who cannot tolerate MRA, or in whom they are contraindicated.

Table 5
ACE inhibitors

Major Guideline Recommendations	AHA/ACC		ESC		CCS		HFSA	
	Class	Level	Class	Level	Class	Level	Class	Level
For patients with current or prior symptoms of HFrEF, to reduce morbidity and mortality	I	A	NS	NS	NS	NS	NS	NS
In addition to a β-blocker, for all patients with an EF ≤40%, to reduce the risk of HF hospitalization and of premature death	NS	NS	I	A	NS	NS	NS	NS
In all symptomatic patients with an EF <40%	NS	NS	NS	NS	Strong	HQ	I	A

Abbreviation: HQ, high quality.

In addition, the CCS and HFSA guidelines recommend ARB as add-on therapy to ACE inhibitors, in cases of intolerance to β-blockers.[4,6,9] This indication is based on subgroup analysis of Val-HeFT, in which showed reduction in the composite end point of morbidity and mortality in patients treated with an ACE inhibitor, but not β-blockers.[21] However, it did not reduce mortality. Key studies include CHARM-Alternative (2003),[26] VALIANT (2003),[27] OPTIMAAL (2002),[28] ELITE II (2000),[29] RESOLVD (1999),[20] Val-HeFT (2001),[21] CHARM-Added (2003).[22]

Mineralocorticoid Receptor Antagonists

Among patients with persisting HF symptoms despite standard therapy, general agreement exists among the guidelines, especially for patients in New York Heart Association (NYHA) class IIIb to IV (**Table 7**). The ESC guidelines recommend MRA for all persistently symptomatic patients (NYHA II–IV).[2] For both the AHA/ACC[9] and CCS guidelines,[4,6] based on the inclusion criteria of the EMPHASIS-HF trial,[23] less symptomatic patients in NYHA class II to IIIa should have a

Table 6
ARBs

Major Guideline Recommendations	AHA/ACC		ESC		CCS		HFSA
	Class	Level	Class	Level	Class	Level	Level
As alternative to an ACE inhibitor because of intolerance (cough or angioedema)	I	A	I	A	Strong	HQ	A
As alternative to an ACE inhibitor as first-line therapy	IIa	A	NS	NS	NS	NS	A (after MI) B (chronic HF)
Persisting symptoms despite standard therapy (ACE inhibitor, β-blocker) ○ As the preferred third drug ○ Unable to tolerate MRA	NS	NS	NS	NS	Strong	MQ	A
Unable to tolerate a β-blocker and have persistent symptoms despite therapy with an ACE inhibitor	NS	NS	NS	NS	Weak	LQ	C

Abbreviation: MRA, mineralocorticoid receptor antagonists.

Table 7
MRAs

Major Guideline Recommendations	AHA/ACC		ESC		CCS		HFSA	
	Class	Level	Class	Level	Class	Level	Class	Level
Persisting symptoms despite standard therapy								
NYHA class II–IIIa	I	A	I	A	Strong	HQ	NS	NS
NYHA class IIIb–IV	I	A	I	A	Strong	HQ	I	A
Following acute MI, LVEF ≤40% with symptoms of HF or DM	I	B	NS	NS	Strong	HQ	IIa	A
Unable to tolerate a β-blocker and have persistent symptoms despite therapy with an ACE inhibitor	NS	NS	NS	NS	NS	NS	IIa	C

+, Recommended with some considerations (see the text).
Abbreviation: DM, diabetes mellitus.

history of prior cardiovascular hospitalization or increased plasma natriuretic peptide levels to be considered for MRA. The HFSA guidelines, published before the trial mentioned earlier, do not formally consider MRA for patients in NYHA class II.[9]

Concerning the use of MRA following MI, there is agreement among the guidelines, although the ESC guidelines do not include it as an official recommendation.[2]

In addition, the recommendation of MRA use in patients unable to tolerate a β-blocker, and with persistent HF symptoms despite therapy with an ACE inhibitor, was stated only by the oldest guideline with a low level of evidence. In any case, these patients are clinically included in the other 2 recommendations. Key studies include RALES (1999),[25] EMPHASIS-HF (2011),[23] and EPHESUS (2003).[24]

β-Blockers

Concerning the use of β-blockers, the main RCTs were performed before 2003. A high degree of agreement in their recommendations is evident among the 4 guidelines. All give a class I-A recommendation for their use in every symptomatic patient with HFrEF (**Table 8**). Terminology for outcomes related to β-blocker use differs between the AHA/ACC, which uses HF hospitalizations and premature death, and the ESC, which uses the less defined terms morbidity and mortality. Although the North American societies just recommend the 3 β-blockers that have been proved

Table 8
β-Blockers

Major Guideline Recommendations	AHA/ACC		ESC		CCS		HFSA	
	Class	Level	Class	Level	Class	Level	Class	Level
For all patients with an EF ≤40%								
In addition to an ACE inhibitor	I	A	I	A	I	A	I	A
Recommended β-blocker:								
One of the 3 proved to reduce mortality	I	A	I	A	Strong	HQ	I	A
Nebivolol	NS	NS	+	+	NS	NS	NS	NS
NYHA class IV patients should be stabilized before starting a β-blocker	NS	NS	NS	NS	Strong	HQ	I	B

Table 9
Digoxin recommendations

Major Guideline Recommendations	AHA/ACC		ESC		CCS		HFSA
	Class	Level	Class	Level	Class	Level	Level
Persisting symptoms despite standard therapy							
NYHA Class II–III	IIa	B	IIb	B	Strong	MQ	NS B
NYHA Class IV	IIa	B	IIb	B	Strong	MQ	C
In patients unable to tolerate a β-blocker	NS	NS	IIb	B	NS	NS	NS NS

to reduce mortality (carvedilol, bisoprolol, and metoprolol XR), the ESC also includes nebivolol, but it clarifies that it has not been shown to reduce cardiovascular or all-cause mortality in patients with HF. In addition, the CCS and HFSA guidelines make an official recommendation regarding initiation of β-blockers only in stabilized patients. Key studies include CIBIS II (1999),[30] MERIT-HF (1999),[31,32] COPERNICUS (2002),[33] SENIORS (2005),[34] and COMET (2003).[35]

Digoxin

Based on the DIG-Trial, all the societies recommend digoxin in patients with HFrEF with persisting symptoms despite standard therapy (**Table 9**). Minor differences exist in the grading of recommendations and in what each society considers standard therapy. Only the ESC guidelines consider the use of digoxin in patients unable to tolerate a β-blocker, which is based on digoxin withdrawal trials during the 1990s (PROVED and RADIANCE). Key studies include DIG (1997),[36] PROVED (1993),[37] and RADIANCE (1993).[38]

Hydralazine and Isosorbide

Clinical use of the combination of hydralazine and isosorbide (HDZ-ISDN) as an alternative to an ACE inhibitors or ARBs, when neither is tolerated or in the presence of contraindications, is recommended by all 4 guidelines (**Table 10**). Each gives a high strength of recommendation, but they differ on the rating of the evidence, which is difficult to understand, considering that it is based on a single RCT (the V-HeFT trial).

Use of HDZ-ISDN combination in patients who remain symptomatic despite ACE inhibitors and β-blockers is also recommended by the 4 guidelines. The AHA/ACC, CCS, and HFSA restrict indication to African American patients, according to the original publication (A-HeFT trial); furthermore, the HFSA gives a higher level of evidence to patients in NYHA class III/IV, because this is the NYHA class of the patients included in this publication. Only the HFSA and ESC guidelines extend this recommendation to nonblack people, reducing the strength of the recommendation and quality of the evidence.

Table 10
Hydralazine and isosorbide

Major Guideline Recommendations	AHA/ACC		ESC		CCS		HFSA	
	Class	Level	Class	Level	Class	Level	Class	Level
As an alternative to an ACE inhibitor or ARB, if neither is tolerated	IIa	B	I	A	Strong	LQ	IIa	C
Persisting symptoms despite standard therapy (ACE inhibitor, B-blocker, MRA)								
In African American patients	I	A	NS	NS	Strong	MQ	I	A/B[a]
In any patient	NS	NS	IIb	B	NS	NS	IIb	C
Unable to tolerate a β-blocker and have persistent symptoms despite therapy with an ACE inhibitor	NS	NS	NS	C	NS	NS	NS	NS

+, Recommended with some considerations (see the text).
[a] Level A for patients in NYHA class III to IV; Level B for patients in NYHA class II.

Use of the HDZ-ISDN combination as add-on therapy to ACE inhibitors in cases of intolerance to β-blockers is recommended only by the HFSA (class C), although there are no studies that directly evaluate the best option in this scenario. Key studies include V-HeFT I (1986),[39] V-HeFT II (1991),[40] and A-HeFT (2004).[41]

Oral Anticoagulants

For chronic anticoagulation in patients with HF with permanent atrial fibrillation (AF), based on classic trials and the CHADS2 (congestive heart failure, hypertension, age ≥75 years, diabetes, prior stroke or transient ischemic attack symptoms) score, AHA/ACC guidelines recommend chronic anticoagulation in patients with HF with 1 additional risk factor for stroke (I- level of evidence A), and make a weaker recommendation if no additional risk factor exists (IIa- level of evidence B).[9] Similarly, the CCS makes a strong recommendation only in patients with high thrombotic risk, according to its own AF guidelines.[4,6] The ESC guidelines, based on more recent trials, recommend chronic anticoagulation if a CHA2DS2-VASC (CHADS2, plus vascular disease, age 65–74 years, sex category) score is greater than or equal to 1,[2] which is the case for patients with coexistent HF and AF. The HFSA also recommends chronic anticoagulation for these patients.

For patients with HF in sinus rhythm and with certain conditions other than AF, the HFSA guidelines, based on old trials, as well as the CCS, recommends anticoagulation (**Table 11**). However, the AHA/ACC does not make any recommendation in these scenarios, although it explicitly recommends avoiding anticoagulation in their absence, based on the futility shown by the newer trials on anticoagulation in HF in sinus rhythm (WASH, WATCH, WARCEF) (key studies include Refs.[42–50]).

NOVEL TREATMENTS
Ivabradine

After the SHIFT trial the ESC made a recommendation for ivabradine in patients in sinus rhythm and a heart rate greater than or equal to 70 beats per minute who are unable to tolerate a β-blocker (IIb, level of evidence C) or persistently symptomatic despite standard therapy (IIa, level of evidence B).[51] No recommendations are available in the other 3 guidelines.

Angiotensin Receptor–Neprilysin Inhibitors

Following the Paradigm Study,[52] the angiotensin receptor–neprilysin inhibitor LCZ696 was recommended by the ESC in patients with mild to moderate HF, an increased natriuretic peptide level, or hospitalization for HF in the past 12 months, in place of an ACE inhibitor or an ARB (conditional, high quality). Only the CCS guidelines (2014 focus update) address the use of LCZ696.

DEVICE RECOMMENDATIONS IN HEART FAILURE
Cardiac Resynchronization Therapy

For patients with NYHA III to IV HF and EF less than or equal to 35%, AHA/ACC criteria are more restrictive than the other guidelines, in terms of QRS morphology and duration (**Table 12**). For example, based on the original COMPANION and CARE-HF trials, the HFSA recommends cardiac resynchronization therapy (CRT) when the QRS length is greater than or equal to 120 milliseconds,

---

Table 11
Oral anticoagulants

Major Guideline Recommendations	AHA/ACC		ESC		CCS		HFSA	
	Class	Level	Class	Level	Class	Level	Class	Level
Patients with HF with chronic AF								
With an additional risk factor for stroke	I	A	NS	NS	Strong	HQ	NS	NS
With no additional risk factor for stroke	IIa	B	I	A	NS	NS	I	A
Patients with HF with conditions other than chronic AF								
Previous systemic embolism	NS	NS	NS	NS	Weak	LQ	I	C
Intracardiac thrombus	NS	NS	NS	NS	Weak	LQ	I	B
After a large anterior MI	NS	NS	NS	NS	Weak	LQ	I	B or C
Patients with HF without AF or special conditions listed above	III	B	NS	NS	Strong	HQ	NS	NS

Table 12
Cardiac resynchronization therapy (CRT)

Major Guideline Recommendations		AHA/ACC		ESC		CCS		HFSA	
QRS Features	EF/NYHA Class	Class	Level	Class	Level	Class	Level	Class	Level
LBBB >150 ms EF <35%									
	Class III-IV	I	A	I	A	Strong	HQ	I/IIb[a]	A/B[a]
	Class II	I	B	—	—	—	—	IIb	C
EF <30%									
	Class II	I	B	I	A	Strong	HQ	IIb	C
120–149 ms EF <35%									
	Class III-IV	IIa	B	I	A	—	—	I/IIb	A/B
	Class II	IIa	B	—	—	—	—	—	—
>130 ms EF <35%									
	Class III-IV	—	—	—	—	Strong	HQ	—	—
EF <30%									
	Class II	—	—	I	A	Strong	HQ	—	—
No LBBB >150 ms EF <35%									
	Class III-IV	IIa	A	IIa	A	Mild	LQ	I/IIb	A/B
	Class II	IIb	B	—	—	—	—	IIb	C
EF <30%									
	Any NYHA class	—	—	IIa	A	Mild	LQ	—	—
120–149 ms EF <35%									
	Class III-IV	IIb	B	—	—	—	—	I/IIb	A/B
	Class II	III	B	—	—	—	—	—	—

Abbreviations: EF, ejection fraction; HQ, high quality; LBBB, left bundle brunch block; LQ, low quality.
[a] Class and Level depends wether the patient is at NYHA III or IV, respectively.

irrespective of morphology (recommendation A). For the ESC guidelines, QRS length must be greater than or equal to 120 milliseconds in the presence of left bundle branch block (LBBB) (I, level of evidence A), and QRS greater than or equal to 150 milliseconds if non-LBBB morphology is present (IIa, level of evidence A). However, The AHA/ACC criteria are more demanding with regard to morphologic criteria, and both QRS greater than or equal to 150 milliseconds and LBBB morphology must coexist for a I- level of evidence A recommendation. For example, patients with EF less than 35%, in NYHA III to IV, QRS greater than or equal to 120 milliseconds, and LBBB morphology have a I- level of evidence A recommendation from the ESC, but are only IIa- level of evidence B in the AHA/ACC guidelines.

For patients with NYHA II HF, the ESC and CCS guidelines are more restrictive than those of the AHA and HFSA in terms of EF. The ESC and CCS guidelines restrict CRT to EF less than 30%, based on the original studies (MADIT-CRT, RAFT), and exclude patients with EF between 30% and 35%, who are included in the HFSA and the AHA guidelines, with a strong recommendation (I- level of evidence B). Regarding QRS width, the HFSA criteria are the strictest, accepting only patients with QRS greater than or equal to 150, but do not incorporate morphologic criteria. This limitation is important, given that CRT in patients in NYHA II has only proved useful in those patients with LBBB morphology, according to a subgroup analysis of MADIT-HF.

The CCS guideline criteria for CRT are similar to those of the ESC, although they incorporate QRS greater than or equal to 130 milliseconds instead of greater than or equal to 120 milliseconds. Despite being published a year before, the guidelines are in alignment with the Echo-CRT trial, which showed increased mortality associated with implantable devices in patients with QRS less than 130 milliseconds. In addition, the strength of the recommendation is lower in non-LBBB morphology.

In patients with a primary clinical need of a pacemaker, CRT should be considered if EF is less than 35% in patients in NYHA class II (IIa-C) or III to IV (I- level of evidence C), independently of the QRS width. In addition, CRT can be useful in patients with AF and EF less than or equal to 35% on guideline-directed medical therapy if (1) the patient requires ventricular pacing or otherwise meets CRT criteria, and (2) atrioventricular nodal ablation or pharmacologic rate control will allow near 100% ventricular pacing with CRT (similar to the AHA/ACC and ESC guidelines). In the HFSA guideline, CRT may be considered for patients with AF, a widened QRS interval (120 milliseconds), and

Table 13
ICD for primary prophylaxis of sudden death

Major Guideline Recommendations	AHA/ACC		ESC		CCS		HFSA	
	Class	Level	Class	Level	Class	Level	Class	Level
Ischemic Cardiomyopathy								
EF <35% NYHA II–III	I	A	I	A	Strong	HQ	I	A
EF <30% NYHA I	I	B	NS	NS	Strong	HQ	NS	NS
EF 31%–35%, irrespective of symptoms	NS	NS	NS	NS	IIa	B	NS	NS
Inducible VF/sustained VT at EPS	NS	NS	NS	NS	IIb	C	NS	NS
No inducible VF/sustained VT at EPS, or without EPS	NS	NS	NS	NS	IIb	C	NS	NS
Nonischemic Cardiomyopathy								
EF <35% NYHA II–III	I	A	I	B	Strong	HQ	I	B
EF <30% NYHA I	I	B	NS	NS	NS	NS	NS	NS

Abbreviations: EPS, electrophysiologic study; VF, ventricular fibrillation; VT, ventricular tachycardia.

LVEF less than 35% who have persistent, moderate to severe HF (NYHA III) despite optimal medical therapy (strength of evidence: B). Key studies include CARE-CRT (2005),[53] the COMPANION Trial (2004),[54] and Echo-CRT (2013)[55] in patients in NYHA FC (Functional Class) III to IV; RAFT (2010) in patients in NYHA FC (Functional Class) II to III[56]; and MADIT-CRT (2009) in patients in NYHA class I to II.[57]

Implantable Cardioverter-Defibrillators for Primary Prevention

All 4 guidelines make strong recommendations on implantable cardioverter-defibrillator (ICD) implantation in patients with HF with EF less than 35%, and in NYHA class II to III, irrespective of cause (ischemic or nonischemic), because these were the inclusion criteria for the pivotal SCD-HeFT trial (**Table 13**). However, in patients with EF less than 30% and in NYHA class I, considerable divergence exists among the societies, which is in part related to the cause of HF. For an ischemic cause, both AHA/ACC and CCS guidelines make strong recommendations, whereas the ESC and HFSA guidelines do not make any statement. For a nonischemic cause, only the AHA/ACC recommends ICD implantation (I- level of evidence B).

Only the CCS includes recommendations for ICD implantation in patients with HF based on electrophysiologic criteria.

Regarding the time requested before ICD implantation, guidelines make different recommendations for ischemic and nonischemic causes. Almost all recommend at least 40 days after MI and more than 3 months following revascularization. In nonischemic causes, optimal medical therapy time requested before ICD implantation is highly variable among guidelines: 3 months according to the ESC, 3 to 6 months according to the HFSA and AHA/ACC (although not incorporated as an specific recommendation), and 6 months according to the CCS (key studies include Refs.[58–60]).

SUMMARY

By comparing these 4 new clinical guidelines in HF from a clinical perspective, this article recognizes that important progress in the approach to diagnosis and treatment of HF has been made in the last 9 years, because more resemblances than important differences were detected among them. In addition, no large gaps are evident regarding methodology for assessing evidence in contemporary clinical definitions of HF. Moreover, among these most influential guidelines, pharmacologic treatments are similar, as are recommendations for CRT and ICDs. A few clinical studies are available regarding emergent new drugs, so further recommendations in the guidelines will follow. Clinical innovation in the management of patients with HF will change these guidelines in the near future.

REFERENCES

1. McMurray J, Swedberg K. Treatment of chronic heart failure: a comparison between the major guidelines. Eur Heart J 2006;33:1787–847.
2. McMurray J, Adamopoulos S, Anker SD, et al. ESC Guidelines for the diagnosis and treatment of acute

and chronic heart failure 2012: The Task Force for the Diagnosis and Treatment of Acute and Chronic Heart Failure 2012 of the European Society of Cardiology. Developed in collaboration with the Heart Failure Association (HFA) of the ESC. Eur Heart J 2012; 27:1773–7.

3. Yancy C, Jessup M, Bozkurt B, et al. 2013 ACCF/AHA guideline for the management of heart failure: executive summary: a report of the American College of Cardiology Foundation/American Heart Association Task Force on practice guidelines. Circulation 2013;128:1810–52.

4. Howlett JG, McKelvie RS, Costigan J, et al. The 2010 Canadian Cardiovascular Society guidelines for the diagnosis and management of heart failure update: heart failure in ethnic minority populations, heart failure and pregnancy, disease management, and quality improvement/assurance programs. Can J Cardiol 2010;26:185–202.

5. McKelvie R, Moe GW, Cheung A, et al. The 2011 Canadian Cardiovascular Society heart failure management guidelines update: focus on sleep apnea, renal dysfunction, mechanical circulatory support, and palliative care. Can J Cardiol 2011;27: 319–38.

6. McKelvie R, Moe GW, Ezekowitz JA, et al. The 2012 Canadian Cardiovascular Society heart failure management guidelines update: focus on acute and chronic heart failure. Can J Cardiol 2013;29: 168–81.

7. Moe GW, Ezekowitz JA, O'Meara E, et al. The 2013 Canadian Cardiovascular Society heart failure management guidelines update: focus on rehabilitation and exercise and surgical coronary revascularization. Can J Cardiol 2014;30:249–63.

8. Moe GW, Ezekowitz JA, O'Meara E, et al. The 2014 Canadian Cardiovascular Society heart failure management guidelines focus update: anemia, biomarkers, and recent therapeutic trial implications. Can J Cardiol 2015;31:3–16.

9. Lindenfeld J, Albert NM, Boehmer JP, et al. HFSA 2010 comprehensive heart failure practice guideline. J Card Fail 2010;16:475–539.

10. The SOLVD Investigators. Effect of enalapril on mortality and the development of heart failure in asymptomatic patients with reduced left ventricular ejection fraction. N Engl J Med 1992;327:685–91.

11. Flather MD, Yusuf S, Kober L, et al. Long-term ACE-inhibitor therapy in patients with heart failure or left-ventricular dysfunction: a systematic overview of data from individual patients. ACE-Inhibitor Myocardial Infarction Collaborative Group. Lancet 2000; 355:1575–81.

12. Dargie HJ. Effect of carvedilol on outcome after myocardial infarction in patients with left-ventricular dysfunction: the CAPRICORN randomized trial. Lancet 2001;357:1385–90.

13. Vantrimpont P, Rouleau JL, Wun CC, et al, SAVE Investigators. Additive beneficial effects of beta-blockers to angiotensin-converting enzyme inhibitors in the Survival and Ventricular Enlargement (SAVE) Study. J Am Coll Cardiol 1997;29:229–36.

14. Exner DV, Dries DL, Waclawiw MA, et al. Beta-adrenergic blocking agent use and mortality in patients with asymptomatic and symptomatic left ventricular systolic dysfunction: a post hoc analysis of the Studies of Left Ventricular Dysfunction. J Am Coll Cardiol 1999;33:916–23.

15. Faris R, Flather M, Purcell H, et al. Current evidence supporting the role of diuretics in heart failure: a meta analysis of randomised controlled trials. Int J Cardiol 2002;82:149–58.

16. Faris R, Flather M, Purcell H, et al. Diuretics for heart failure. Cochrane Database Syst Rev 2012;(2): CD003838.

17. Effects of enalapril on mortality in severe congestive heart failure. Results of the Cooperative North Scandinavian Enalapril Survival Study (CONSENSUS). The CONSENSUS Trial Study Group. N Engl J Med 1987;316:1429–35.

18. Effect of enalapril on survival in patients with reduced left ventricular ejection fractions and congestive heart failure. The SOLVD Investigators. N Engl J Med 1991;325:293–302.

19. Packer M, Poole-Wilson P, Armstrong P, et al. Comparative effects of low and high doses of the angiotensin-converting enzyme inhibitor, lisinopril, on morbidity and mortality in chronic heart failure. ATLAS Study Group. Circulation 1999;100:2312–8.

20. McKelvie R, Yusuf S, Pericak D, et al. Comparison of candesartan, enalapril, and their combination in congestive heart failure: Randomized Evaluation of Strategies for Left Ventricular Dysfunction (RESOLVD) pilot study. The RESOLVD Pilot Study Investigators. Circulation 1999;100:1056.

21. Cohn J, Tognoni G, Valsartan Heart Failure Trial Investigators. A randomized trial of the angiotensin-receptor blocker valsartan in chronic heart failure. N Engl J Med 2001;345:1667.

22. McMurray J, Ostergren J, Swedberg K, et al. Effects of candesartan in patients with chronic heart failure and reduced left-ventricular systolic function taking angiotensin-converting-enzyme inhibitors: the CHARM-Added trial. Lancet 2003;362:767.

23. Zannad F, McMurray J, Krum H, et al. Eplerenone in patients with systolic heart failure and mild symptoms. N Engl J Med 2011;364:11–21.

24. Pitt B, Remme W, Zannad F, et al. Eplerenone, a selective aldosterone blocker, in patients with left ventricular dysfunction after myocardial infarction. N Engl J Med 2003;348:1309–21.

25. Pitt B, Zannad F, Remme W, et al. The effect of spironolactone on morbidity and mortality in patients with severe heart failure. Randomized Aldactone

Evaluation Study Investigators. N Engl J Med 1999; 341:709–17.

26. Granger C, McMurray J, Yusuf S, et al. Effects of candesartan in patients with chronic heart failure and reduced left-ventricular systolic function intolerant to angiotensin-converting-enzyme inhibitors: the CHARM-Alternative trial. Lancet 2003;362:772.

27. Pfeffer M, Mc Murray J, Velazquez E, et al. Valsartan, captopril, or both in myocardial infarction complicated by heart failure, left ventricular dysfunction, or both. N Engl J Med 2003;349:1893.

28. Dickstein K, Kjekshus J. Effects of losartan and captopril on mortality and morbidity in high-risk patients after acute myocardial infarction: the OPTIMAAL randomized trial. Optimal Trial in Myocardial Infarction with Angiotensin II Antagonist Losartan. Lancet 2002;3(60):752–60.

29. Pitt B, Poole-Wilson P, Segal R, et al. Effect of losartan compared with captopril on mortality in patients with symptomatic heart failure: randomised trial—the Losartan Heart Failure Survival Study ELITE II. Lancet 2000;355:1582–7.

30. The Cardiac Insufficiency Bisoprolol Study II (CIBIS-II): a randomised trial. Lancet 1999;353:9–13.

31. Effect of metoprolol CR/XL in chronic heart failure: Metoprolol CR/XL Randomised Intervention Trial in Congestive Heart Failure (MERIT-HF). Lancet 1999; 353:2001–7.

32. Hjalmarson A, Goldstein S, Fagerberg B, et al. Effects of controlled-release metoprolol on total mortality, hospitalizations, and well-being in patients with heart failure: the Metoprolol CR/XL Randomized Intervention Trial in congestive heart failure (MERIT-HF). MERIT-HF Study Group. JAMA 2000;283: 1295–302.

33. Packer M, Fowler M, Roecker E, et al. Effect of carvedilol on the morbidity of patients with severe chronic heart failure: results of the carvedilol prospective randomized cumulative survival (COPERNICUS) study. Circulation 2002;106:2194–9.

34. Flather M, Shibata M, Coats A, et al. Randomized trial to determine the effect of nebivolol on mortality and cardiovascular hospital admission in elderly patients with heart failure (SENIORS). Eur Heart J 2005; 26:215–25.

35. Poole-Wilson P, Swedberg K, Cleland J, et al. Comparison of carvedilol and metoprolol on clinical outcomes in patients with chronic heart failure in the Carvedilol Or Metoprolol European Trial (COMET): randomised controlled trial. Lancet 2003;362:7–13.

36. Digitalis Investigation Group. The effect of digoxin on mortality and morbidity in patients with heart failure. N Engl J Med 1997;336:525.

37. Uretsky B, Young J, Shahidi F, et al. Randomized study assessing the effect of digoxin withdrawal in patients with mild to moderate chronic congestive heart failure: results of the PROVED trial. PROVED Investigative Group. J Am Coll Cardiol 1993;22:955.

38. Packer M, Gheorghiade M, Young J, et al. Withdrawal of digoxin from patients with chronic heart failure treated with angiotensin-converting-enzyme inhibitors. RADIANCE Study. N Engl J Med 1993;329:1.

39. Cohn J, Archibald D, Ziesche S, et al, for the Veterans Administration Cooperative Study Group. Effect of vasodilator therapy on mortality in chronic congestive heart failure. Results of a Veterans Administration Cooperative Study. N Engl J Med 1986;314:1547–52.

40. Cohn JN, Johnson G, Ziesche S. A comparison of enalapril with hydralazine–isosorbide dinitrate in the treatment of chronic congestive heart failure. N Engl J Med 1991;325:303–10.

41. Taylor A, Ziesche S, Yancy C, et al. Combination of isosorbide dinitrate and hydralazine in blacks with heart failure. N Engl J Med 2004;351:2049–57.

42. Risk factors for stroke and efficacy of antithrombotic therapy in atrial fibrillation: analysis of pooled data from five randomized controlled trials. Arch Intern Med 1994;154:1449–57 [Erratum appears in Arch Intern Med 1994;154:2254].

43. Hughes M, Lip G. Stroke and thromboembolism in atrial fibrillation: a systematic review of stroke risk factors, risk stratification schema and cost effectiveness data. Thromb Haemost 2008;99:295–304.

44. Lip G, Nieuwlaat R, Pisters R, et al. Refining clinical risk stratification for predicting stroke and thromboembolism in atrial fibrillation using a novel risk factor-based approach: the Euro Heart Survey on atrial fibrillation. Chest 2010;137:263–72.

45. Kyrle P, Korninger C, Gossinger H, et al. Prevention of arterial and pulmonary embolism by oral anticoagulants in patients with dilated cardiomyopathy. Thromb Haemost 1985;54:521–3.

46. Ciaccheri M, Castelli G, Cecchi F, et al. Lack of correlation between intracavitary thrombosis detected by cross sectional echocardiography and systemic emboli in patients with dilated cardiomyopathy. Br Heart J 1989;62:26–9.

47. Dunkman W, Johnson G, Carson P, et al. Incidence of thromboembolic events in congestive heart failure. The V-HeFT VA Cooperative Studies Group. Circulation 1993;87:VI94–101.

48. Cleland J, Findlay I, Jafri S, et al. The Warfarin/Aspirin Study in Heart failure (WASH): a randomized trial comparing antithrombotic strategies for patients with heart failure. Am Heart J 2004;148: 157–64.

49. Massie B, Collins J, Ammon S, et al. Randomized trial of warfarin, aspirin, and clopidogrel in patients with chronic heart failure: the Warfarin and

Antiplatelet Therapy in Chronic Heart Failure (WATCH) trial. Circulation 2009;119:1616–24.

50. Homma S, Thompson J, Pullicino P, et al. Warfarin and aspirin in patients with heart failure and sinus rhythm. N Engl J Med 2012;366:1859–69.

51. Swedberg K, Komajda M, Bohm M, et al. Ivabradine and outcomes in chronic heart failure (SHIFT): a randomised placebo-controlled study. Lancet 2010;376:875–85.

52. McMurray J, Packer M, Desai A, et al. Angiotensin-neprilysin inhibition versus enalapril in heart failure. N Engl J Med 2014;371:993.

53. Cleland JG, Daubert JC, Erdmann E, et al. The effect of cardiac resynchronization on morbidity and mortality in heart failure. N Engl J Med 2005;352:1539 (CARE).

54. Bristow MR, Saxon LA, Boehmer J, et al. Cardiac-resynchronization therapy with or without an implantable defibrillator in advanced chronic heart failure. N Engl J Med 2004;350:2140 (COMPANION).

55. Ruschitzka F, Abraham WT, Singh JP, et al. Cardiac-resynchronization therapy in heart failure with a narrow QRS complex. N Engl J Med 2013;369: 1395 (Echo-CRT).

56. Tang AS, Wells GA, Talajic M, et al. Cardiac-resynchronization therapy for mild-to-moderate heart failure. N Engl J Med 2010;363:2385 (RAFT).

57. Moss AJ, Hall WJ, Cannom DS, et al. Cardiac-resynchronization therapy for the prevention of heart-failure events. N Engl J Med 2009;361:1329.

58. Bardy GH, Lee KL, Mark DB, et al. Amiodarone or an implantable cardioverter-defibrillator for congestive heart failure. N Engl J Med 2005;352:225–37.

59. Moss AJ, Hall WJ, Cannom DS, et al. Improved survival with an implanted defibrillator in patients with coronary disease at high risk for ventricular arrhythmia. Multicenter Automatic Defibrillator Implantation Trial Investigators. N Engl J Med 1996;335:1933–40.

60. Kadish A, Dyer A, Daubert JP, et al. Prophylactic defibrillator implantation in patients with nonischemic dilated cardiomyopathy. N Engl J Med 2004; 350:2151–8.

Prognostic Factors in Hospitalization for Heart Failure in Asia

 CrossMark

Seok-Min Kang, MD, PhD[a], Myeong-Chan Cho, MD, PhD[b],*

KEYWORDS

- Heart failure • Hospitalization • Prognostic factors

KEY POINTS

- The prevalence of heart failure (HF) with repeated rehospitalization because of worsening of HF is increasing and becoming a critical economic burden in Asian countries.
- Each hospitalization is associated with progressive myocardial or renal injuries that cause a high rehospitalization rate and postdischarge mortality.
- Various clinical characteristics, causes, and treatment strategies may account for the differences in the prognostic factors for clinical outcomes between Asian countries.
- Periodic HF registries leading to better understanding of the characteristics of Asian patients hospitalized with HF are warranted in the future.

INTRODUCTION

Heart failure (HF) is a complex clinical syndrome and a global public health problem that is a leading cause of hospitalization because of repeated worsening of HF. Thus, recurrent rehospitalization is becoming a critical issue with a growing economic burden in Asian countries. Furthermore, patients hospitalized with HF have a higher postdischarge mortality with higher rehospitalization rates.[1] Despite recent advances in the management of HF, the prevalence of HF is steadily increasing all over the world because of the increased risk factors of HF, increased aging population, and better survival after cardiovascular events. The population of Asia is growing both larger and older. People aged 65 years and older will make up an increasingly large percentage of the Asian population in future years, especially in Korea and Japan.

Although the mortality of HF may have begun to decline over recent years, the rehospitalization rate has remained unchanged, and may even get worse in the United States and several European countries.[2–4] According to Western data, postdischarge mortality and the rehospitalization rate reach up to 20% and 30%, respectively, within 6 months.

Hospitalization with HF (HHF) is characterized by rapid worsening of chronic HF or new-onset (de novo) acute HF requiring urgent therapy, accompanied by electrolyte imbalance, neurohormonal activation, renal impairment, and hemodynamic alterations. HHF can be divided into HF with reduced ejection fraction (HFrEF) and HF with preserved ejection fraction (HFpEF). Most patients hospitalized with HF have symptoms and signs of volume overload, rather than low cardiac output.[5]

Previous observational large-scale HHF cohort studies and surveys from Western countries, such as the Acute Decompensated Heart Failure National Registry (ADHERE)[6], the Organized Program to

Conflicts of interest: None.
[a] Cardiology Division, Severance Cardiovascular Hospital and Cardiovascular Research Institute, Yonsei University College of Medicine, Seoul, Korea; [b] Cardiology Division, Department of Internal Medicine, College of Medicine, Chungbuk National University, 776 Sunhwan-1-Ro, Seowon-Gu, Cheongju 362-711, Korea
* Corresponding author.
E-mail address: mccho@chungbuk.ac.kr

Heart Failure Clin 11 (2015) 543–550
http://dx.doi.org/10.1016/j.hfc.2015.07.006
1551-7136/15/$ – see front matter © 2015 Elsevier Inc. All rights reserved.

Initiate Lifesaving Treatment in Hospitalized Patients With Heart Failure (OPTIMIZE-HF) in the United States, and EuroHeart Failure Survey II (EHFS II) in Europe, have identified several prognostic factors in hospitalized patients with HF.[7,8] The widely accepted prognostic factors include age, low blood pressure, ischemic heart disease, a reduced left ventricular (LV) function, hyponatremia, and renal dysfunction. However, prognostic factors for clinical outcomes in hospitalized patients with HF may not be similar in Asian people, because of different clinical characteristics, causes, and treatment responses or strategies according to different medical cultures and health care systems.

This article provides an overview of the current or emerging clinical and biological prognostic factors in Asian HHF registries (**Table 1**), including KorHF[9] (Korean Heart Failure) registry and KorAHF[10] (Korean Acute Heart Failure) registry in Korea, JCARE-CARD[11,12] (Japanese Cardiac Registry of Heart Failure in Cardiology) registry and ATTEND[13,14] (The Acute Decompensated Heart Failure Syndromes) registry in Japan, and ADHERE International–AP[15] (Acute Decompensated Heart Failure Registry—Asia-Pacific) registry in Asia-Pacific countries, with a viewpoint to developing a treatment strategy that will improve the management of hospitalized patients with HF in Asia.

PROGNOSTIC FACTORS OF MORTALITY AND MORBIDITY

Recent Asian registries for HF have identified prognostic factors in hospitalized patients with HF (**Table 2**).

Age

HF is one of the leading causes of death and hospitalization in elderly patients. Age was considered to be one of predictors of all-cause mortality in the KorHF registry in both univariate (hazard ratio [HR], 1.027; 95% confidence interval, 1.021–1.034; $P<.001$) and multivariate analysis (HR, 1.023; 95% confidence interval, 1.004–1.042; $P = .020$).[9] According to KorAHF data, old age ($\geq$70 years) was an independent predictor of postdischarge mortality.[10] The JCARE-CARD data showed that all-cause death (36.6% vs 14.7%), cardiac death (23.2% vs 8.8%), and rehospitalization (45% vs 33.1%) were significantly higher in hospitalized patients with HF older than 80 years compared with patients aged less than 80 years.[16] Presumably, these findings are related to older patients with HF having multiple comorbidities with high risk factors and less received evidence-based medical or device therapy compared with young patients.

Table 1 HHF registries in Asian countries	
KorHF Registry[9]	Nationwide, prospective, observational, multicenter registry from 24 academic hospitals for hospitalized Korean patients with acute HF, between June 2004 and April 2009 (n = 3200)
KorAHF Registry[10]	Nationwide, prospective, observational, multicenter cohort registry from 10 tertiary university hospitals for hospitalized Korean patients with acute HF, funded by the Korea National Institute of Health, between March 2011 and December 2013 (n = 5766)
JCARE-CARD Registry[11,12]	National prospective registry from 164 teaching hospitals for hospitalized patients with acute HF in Japan, between January 2004 and June 2005 (n = 2675)
ATTEND Registry[13,14]	Nationwide, multicenter, patient-based, prospective, observational cohort registry involving 53 medical hospitals for hospitalized patients with acute HF throughout Japan, between April 2007 and December 2011 (n = 4842)
ADHERE International Asia-Pacific Registry[15]	Multicenter, observational registry from 43 hospitals for hospitalized patients with acute decompensated HF in 8 Asia-Pacific countries, between January 2006 and December 2008 (n = 10,171), including 29% from Singapore, 20% from Thailand, 17% from Indonesia, 8.9% from Australia, 8.9% from Malaysia, 7.1% from the Philippines, 5.3% from Taiwan, and 3.9% from Hong Kong

Abbreviations: ADHERE, Acute Decompensated Heart Failure National Registry; ATTEND, Acute Decompensated Heart Failure Syndromes; JCARE-CARD, Japanese Cardiac Registry of Heart Failure in Cardiology; KorAHF, Korean Acute Heart Failure; KorHF, Korean Heart Failure.

Table 2
Reported prognostic factors and emerging targets in Asian hospitalized patients with HF

Age	Advanced age is an independent predictor of postdischarge mortality and rehospitalization[9,10,16]
Hyponatremia	Up to 25% in Asian HHF Associated with in-hospital mortality and postdischarge mortality[9,10,14,17,18]
SBP	Low admission SBP is associated with higher in-hospital mortality[9,10,12,14,20]
Renal dysfunction	One of the most important poor prognostic factors of in-hospital mortality and postdischarge mortality[9,10,22,23]
Left ventricular function	No significant difference in in-hospital and long-term mortality between patients with HFrEF and HFpEF[24]
Ventricular conduction disturbance	Prolonged QRS duration occurs in approximately 20%, with a significant poor predictor of all-cause mortality and rehospitalization, particularly in patients with LV systolic dysfunction RBBB was an independent predictor of in-hospital mortality[26,27]
Anemia	Anemia at admission is associated with all-cause death and repeated hospitalization 8.9% increase in all-cause death or rehospitalization for each 1-g/dL decrease in discharge hemoglobin level after discharge[9,28–30]
Evidence-based medication adherence	Adherence to evidence-based medicine at discharge is associated with improved clinical outcomes in patients with reduced systolic dysfunction[12,32]
Emerging and other targets	Hemoconcentration, soluble ST2, NGAL, copeptin, galectin-3, BNP/NT-proBNP, CRP, and RDW[36,37,39]

Abbreviations: BNP, brain natriuretic peptide; CRP, C-reactive protein; NGAL, neutrophil gelatinase–associated lipocalin; NT-proBNP, N-terminal pro–brain natriuretic peptide; RBBB, right bundle branch block; RDW, red cell distribution width; SBP, systolic blood pressure.

Hyponatremia

Hyponatremia, defined as a serum sodium concentration less than 135 mEq/L, predicts poor prognosis in hospitalized patients with HF in Western countries. It is a common finding, irrespective of systolic function, with an incidence of up to 25% in hospitalized Asian patients with HF. Data from the KorHF registry in Korea showed that hyponatremia at admission was associated with higher all-cause mortality, irrespective of whether hyponatremia improves during hospitalization.[17] The interim analysis of KorAHF registry data showed that hyponatremia at admission was an independent predictor of in-hospital mortality and postdischarge mortality in multivariate regression analysis.[10] The JCARE-CARD registry found that hyponatremia at admission was a predictor of in-hospital mortality and long-term mortality.[14]

Also, the ATTEND registry in Japan showed that hospitalized hyponatremic patients with HF required more intensive care because of their more critical condition, with a poorer prognosis (much higher in-hospital mortality of 11.4% in hyponatremic patients compared with 3.6% in normonatremic patients).[18] Thus, hyponatremia at admission is an important prognostic factor in hospitalized Asian patients with HF.

Although the Efficacy of Vasopressin Antagonism in Heart Failure Outcome Study With Tolvaptan (EVEREST) trial,[19] in which tolvaptan effectively correct hyponatremia, could not show improved clinical outcomes in hospitalized Western patients with HF, including only 8% with hyponatremia, a large prospective study using a vasopressin antagonists should be conducted in hospitalized Asian patients with HF with hyponatremia.

Systolic Blood Pressure

In general, the systolic blood pressure (SBP) of patients with HFrEF is lower than that of patients with HFpEF. The ATTEND registry in Japan showed that admission SBP of less than 120 mm Hg was observed more in patients with HFrEF than in patients with HFpEF.[20]

It has been reported that SBP on admission and early after discharge is associated with in-hospital and postdischarge mortality, respectively, in hospitalized patients with HF. A higher SBP inversely correlates with a lower in-hospital and postdischarge mortality.[21] In several Asian HF registries, SBP on admission has been shown to be an important prognostic factor for in-hospital and postdischarge mortality. According to the data from the Korean registries, low SBP (<120 mm Hg in KorHF and <100 mm Hg in KorAHF) was a predictor for all-cause mortality and in-hospital mortality.[9,10] The JCARE-CARD registry found SBP less than 110 mm Hg to be a predictor of in-hospital mortality.[12] The ATTEND registry showed that low SBP (<100 mm Hg) on admission was associated with an extremely high in-hospital mortality (20%).[14]

Renal Dysfunction

Renal dysfunction is one of the most important findings during hospitalization and prognostic factors in hospitalized patients with HF. Recent studies have shown that renal dysfunction is more related to systemic venous congestion than low cardiac output. Of the ATTEND registry data, renal dysfunction (defined as estimated glomerular filtration rate [eGFR] ≤ 50 mL/min/1.73 m^2 using the modification of diet in renal disease [MDRD] equation) was present in 49.8%. Patients with renal dysfunction had a significant in-hospital mortality (odds ratio, 2.36; 95% confidence interval, 1.75–3.18; $P<.001$), irrespective of clinical hemodynamic profiles.[22] However, in the KorHF registry data, renal dysfunction (creatinine [Cr] level ≥ 2.0 mg/dL) is associated with poor clinical outcomes only in univariate analysis, but not in multivariate analysis.[9] The KorAHF registry showed that Cr level greater than or equal to 2.0 mg/dL at admission was one of the most important poor prognostic factors of in-hospital mortality and postdischarge mortality in multivariate regression analysis.[10] Oh and colleagues[23] showed that estimation of glomerular filtration rate using new Chronic Kidney Disease Epidemiology Collaboration (CKD-EPI) equation would have a better prognostic power than the MDRD equation in the prediction of clinical outcomes in hospitalized Korean patients with HF. More accurate estimation of renal dysfunction using CKD-EPI equation might result in improved risk stratification in hospitalized Asian patients with HF.

Left Ventricular Function

The OPTIMIZE-HF study showed that postdischarge event rate and mortality were similar between patients with HFrEF and patients with HFpEF.[7] Consistent with Western results, the data from the JCARE-CARD registry showed that in-hospital as well as long-term mortality, such as all-cause, cardiovascular mortality, and rate of rehospitalization because of worsening of HF, were not significantly different between patients with HFrEF and patients with HFpEF.[24]

Ventricular Conduction Disturbance

Prolonged QRS duration (>120 milliseconds) has been known to be a poor prognostic factor in patients with chronic HF. However, there is little information regarding the prognostic implication of QRS duration in hospitalized patients with HF.[25] The KorHF registry data show that prolonged QRS duration is present in 19.9%, with a significant poor predictor of all-cause mortality and rehospitalization, particularly in those with LV systolic dysfunction.[26] Inconsistent data exist regarding the prognostic role of bundle branch block (BBB) patterns for clinical outcomes in hospitalized patients with HF. Based on KorHF data, right BBB (RBBB) was present in 5.4%, left BBB (LBBB) in 4.9%, and no BBB in 89.7%. RBBB, not LBBB, was associated with higher all-cause mortality and rehospitalization, especially in those with reduced LV systolic function.[27] Also, the KorAHF data showed that RBBB was an independent predictor of in-hospital mortality.[10] The prognostic significance of prolonged QRS duration or BBB pattern in hospitalized patients with HFpEF should be investigated.

Anemia

Anemia (hemoglobin [Hb] level <13 g/dL for men, and <12 g/dL for women) is a well-known predictor of poor prognosis in chronic ambulatory HF and is commonly observed in hospitalized patients with HF as well. The KorHF registry showed that anemia on admission was an independent predictor for all-cause mortality in hospitalized patients with HF.[9] The JCARE-CARD registry found anemia (Hb level <10 g/dL) on admission to be a predictor of long-term mortality. Also, there was an 8.9% increase in all-cause death or rehospitalization for each 1-g/dL decrease in discharge Hb concentration ($P<.001$) during the 2.4-year follow-up after hospital discharge.[28] The ATTEND registry found that all-cause death and the composite outcome of all-cause death and readmission for HF were significantly higher in patients with anemia than in those without anemia. Subgroup analysis of the prognostic value of anemia revealed that anemia on admission was associated with higher all-cause mortality in patients who were aged less than 75 years, male, had new-onset HF, and had HFrEF.[29] However, Hong and colleagues[30] suggested that, in hospitalized Korean patients with HF with severe renal dysfunction (eGFR<45 mL/min/1.73 m^2), admission anemia was not an independent predictor of cardiovascular mortality and rehospitalization. New-onset anemia (defined as presence of anemia at 1 month after discharge without the evidence of anemia) was significantly associated with higher cardiovascular mortality and morbidity in these patients.

Evidence-based Medication Adherence

Current data show that all-cause mortality and re-hospitalization after discharge of hospitalized patients with HF were higher during the first month after discharge compared with other cardiovascular diseases, such as acute myocardial infarction. Although current American College of Cardiology/American Heart Association guidelines[31] recommend performance measures before discharge in hospitalized patients with HF to improve clinical outcomes, few data about adherence to performance measures and the effect on clinical outcomes of hospitalized patients with HF in Korea and other Asian countries were reported. Youn and colleagues[32] showed that adherence to prescription of angiotensin-converting enzyme inhibitors/angiotensin receptor II blockers (ARBs) and β-blocker use at discharge are associated with improved clinical outcomes in hospitalized patients with HF with LV systolic dysfunction (ejection fraction <40%). The data from JCARE-CARD showed that ARB use before admission was related to lower in-hospital mortality.[12] Because the guideline-directed medical therapy has been shown to improve clinical outcomes of hospitalized patients with HF, a tailored approach including a management strategy to promote adherence to clinical guidelines was needed in hospitalized Asian patients with HF.

Hospitalization

Recently, hospitalization for worsening of HF has itself been recognized as one of the most important prognostic factors of postdischarge mortality and rehospitalization in hospitalized patients with HF. With each hospitalization, myocardial injury, which may be related to a decrease in coronary perfusion and/or further activation of neurohormones and renal dysfunction, probably contributes to progressive myocardial or renal dysfunction, leading to short-term and postdischarge morbidity and mortality (**Fig. 1**).[33]

Considering Asian lifestyles, such as large families, repeated rehospitalization of HF is a growing financial problem, especially in elderly patients who need to be looked after. Therefore, early recognition and treatment of prognostic factors in hospitalized patients with HF might improve postdischarge survival and prevent rehospitalization, which are the most important goals in the management of patients with HF.

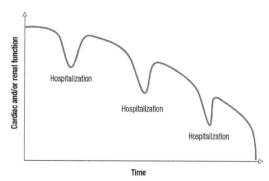

Fig. 1. Each rehospitalization contributes to progressive myocardial or renal dysfunction, leading to short-term and postdischarge morbidity and mortality. (*Adapted from* Gheorghiade M, De Luca L, Fonarow GC, et al. Pathophysiologic targets in the early phase of acute heart failure syndromes. Am J Cardiol 2005;96(Suppl):11G–7G; with permission.)

EMERGING PROGNOSTIC FACTORS
Hemoconcentration

Hemoconcentration, defined as increasing Hb and/or hematocrit levels during hospitalization, is considered to be a surrogate marker that predicts effective diuresis, and is associated with improved survival in hospitalized patients with HF, even in the setting of worsening of renal function.[34,35] Consistent with the results from hospitalized Western patients with HF, the study based on the KorHF registry shows that hemoconcentration during hospitalization is a good prognostic marker of all-cause mortality and HF rehospitalization, independent of the presence of anemia at admission. Also, there is a linear trend in clinical outcomes related to the degree of hemoconcentration.[36] Therefore, prospective randomized trials of decongestive strategies based on hemoconcentration would be interesting in the risk stratification of hospitalized patients with HF.

OTHER PROGNOSTIC FACTORS

Other prognostic markers, such as plasma norepinephrine, plasma renin activity, vasopressin, cardiac troponin, brain natriuretic peptide (BNP), N-terminal pro-BNP (NT-proBNP), C-reactive protein (CRP), soluble ST2, neutrophil gelatinase–associated lipocalin (NGAL), copeptin, and galectin-3 seem to be associated with increased postdischarge mortality in hospitalized patients with HF. Among them, analysis of the KorHF registry data showed that both increase of high-sensitivity CRP as a marker for inflammation and NT-proBNP as a marker for neurohumoral activation were independently associated with 1-year mortality. Furthermore, combination of both markers predicts better prognostic discrimination for clinical outcomes in hospitalized Korean patients with HF.[37] Recently, red cell distribution width (RDW), both at admission and at discharge, has been shown to be a novel prognostic marker independently associated with adverse outcomes in acute HF.[38] Oh and colleagues[39] showed that positive change of RDW between admission and 1 month after discharge was an independent prognostic factor for cardiovascular mortality and rehospitalization, although their study was performed in a single center with a small number of hospitalized patients with HF. However, simple, inexpensive, repeated measurement of RDW may assist in determining risk stratification in hospitalized patients with HF.

However, there is no evidence for the prognostic role of new biomarkers such as soluble ST2, NGAL, copeptin, and galectin-3 in hospitalized Asian patients with HF. However, a clinical multimarker approach or serial biomarker measurement may have a greater predictability in determining the prognosis of hospitalized patients with HF.

SUMMARY

The HHF population is becoming a significant economic burden to Asian countries, because of the growing elderly population, increased prevalence of HF, and recurrent rehospitalization. A targeted treatment strategy is therefore needed with prognostic factors that can reduce the mortality or rehospitalization rate after discharge in these patients. Many epidemiologic studies have attempted to find prognostic factors for clinical outcomes in hospitalized Asian patients with HF, but conflicting results are reported. There are ethnic variations for the differences in the causes, management, and clinical outcomes of hospitalized Asian patients with HF. Further research leading to better understanding of the characteristics of hospitalized Asian patients with HF is warranted.

REFERENCES

1. Ambrosy AP, Fonarow GC, Butler J, et al. The global health and economic burden of hospitalization for heart failure: lessons learned from hospitalized heart failure registries. J Am Coll Cardiol 2014;63: 1123–33.
2. Blecker S, Paul LM, Taksler G, et al. Heart failure associated hospitalizations in the United States. J Am Coll Cardiol 2013;61:1259–67.
3. Schaufelberger M, Swedberg K, Koster M, et al. Decreasing one-year mortality and hospitalization rates for heart failure in Sweden; data from the Swedish Hospital Discharge Registry 1988 to 2000. Eur Heart J 2004;25:300–7.
4. Stewart S, MacIntyre K, MacLeod MM, et al. Trends in hospitalization for heart failure in Scotland, 1990–1996. An epidemic that has reached its peak? Eur Heart J 2001;22:209–17.
5. Gheorghiade M, Pang PS. Acute heart failure syndromes. J Am Coll Cardiol 2009;53:557–73.
6. Adams KF Jr, Fonarow GC, Emerman CL, et al. Characteristics and outcomes of patients hospitalized for heart failure in the United States: rationale, design, and preliminary observations from the first 100,000 cases in the Acute Decompensated Heart Failure National Registry (ADHERE). Am Heart J 2005;149:209–16.
7. Abraham WT, Fonarow GC, Albert NM, et al. Predictors of in-hospital mortality in patients hospitalized for heart failure: insight from the Organized Program to Initiate Lifesaving Treatment in Hospitalized Patients With Heart Failure (OPTIMIZE-HF). J Am Coll Cardiol 2008;52:347–56.
8. Komajda M, Hanon O, Hochadel M, et al. Contemporary management of octogenarians hospitalized for heart failure in Europe: Euro Heart Failure Survey II. Eur Heart J 2009;30:478–86.
9. Choi DJ, Han S, Jeon ES, et al. Characteristics, outcomes and predictors of long-term mortality for patients hospitalized for acute heart failure: a report from the Korean Heart Failure Registry. Korean Circ J 2011;41:363–71.
10. Lee SE, Cho HJ, Lee HY, et al. A multicenter cohort study of acute heart failure syndromes in Korea: rationale, design, and interim observations of the Korean Acute Heart Failure (KorAHF) registry. Eur J Heart Fail 2014;16:700–8.
11. Tsutsui H, Tsuchihashi-Makaya M, Kinugawa S, et al. Clinical characteristics and outcome of hospitalized patients with heart failure in Japan: rationale and design of Japanese Cardiac Registry of Heart Failure in Cardiology (JCARE-CARD). Circ J 2006;70: 1617–23.
12. Hamaguchi S, Kinugawa S, Tsuchihashi-Makaya M, et al. Characteristics, management, and outcomes for patients during hospitalization due to worsening heart failure-A report from the Japanese Cardiac Registry of Heart Failure in Cardiology (JCARE-CARD). J Cardiol 2013;62:95–101.
13. Sato N, Kajimoto K, Asai K, et al. Acute decompensated heart failure syndromes (ATTEND) Registry. A prospective observational multicenter cohort study: rationale, design, and preliminary data. Am Heart J 2010;159:949–55.
14. Sato N, Kajimoto K, Keida T, et al. Clinical features and outcome in hospitalized heart failure in Japan (from the ATTEND Registry). Circ J 2013; 77:944–51.

15. Atherton JJ, Hayward CS, Ahmad WA, et al. Patient characteristics from a regional multicenter database of acute decompensated heart failure in Asia-Pacific (ADHERE International-Asia Pacific). J Card Fail 2012;18:82–8.

16. Hamaguchi S, Kinugawa S, Goto D, et al. Predictors of long-term adverse outcomes in elderly patients over 80 years hospitalized with heart failure - A report from the Japanese Cardiac Registry of Heart Failure in Cardiology (JCARE-CARD). Circ J 2011;75:2403–10.

17. Lee SE, Choi DJ, Yoon CH, et al. Improvement of hyponatremia during hospitalization for acute heart failure is not associated with improvement of prognosis: an analysis from the Korean Heart Failure (KorHF) registry. Heart 2012;98:1798–804.

18. Sato N, Gheorghiade M, Kajimoto K, et al. Hyponatremia and in-hospital mortality in patients admitted for heart failure (from the ATTEND Registry). Am J Cardiol 2013;111:1019–25.

19. Konstam MA, Gheorghiade M, Burnett JC Jr, et al. Efficacy of Vasopressin Antagonism in Heart Failure Outcome Study with Tolvaptan (EVEREST) Investigators. Effects of oral tolvaptan in patients hospitalized for worsening heart failure. The EVEREST Outcome trial. JAMA 2007;297:1319–31.

20. Kajimoto K, Sato N, Sakata Y, et al. Relationship between systolic blood pressure and preserved or reduced ejection fraction at admission in patients hospitalized for acute heart failure syndromes. Int J Cardiol 2013;168:4790–5.

21. Gheorghiade M, Abraham WT, Albert NM, et al. Systolic blood pressure at admission, clinical characteristics, and outcomes in patients hospitalized with acute heart failure. JAMA 2006;296:2217–26.

22. Inohara T, Kohsaka S, Sato N, et al. Prognostic impact of renal dysfunction does not differ according to the clinical profiles of patients: insight from the Acute Decompensated Heart Failure Syndromes (ATTEND) Registry. PLoS One 2014;9:1–8.

23. Oh J, Kang SM, Hong N, et al. The CKD-EPI is more accurate in clinical outcome prediction than MDRD equation in acute heart failure: data from the Korean Heart Failure (KorHF) Registry. Int J Cardiol 2013;167:1084–7.

24. Tsuchihashi-Makaya M, Hamaguchi S, Kinugawa S, et al. Characteristics and outcomes of hospitalized patients with heart failure and reduced vs preserved ejection fraction - A report from the Japanese Cardiac Registry of Heart Failure in Cardiology (JCARE-CARD). Circ J 2009;73:1893–900.

25. Wang NC, Maggioni AP, Konstam MA, et al. Clinical implications of QRS duration in patients hospitalized with worsening heart failure and reduced left ventricular ejection fraction. JAMA 2008;299:2656–66.

26. Park HS, Kim H, Park JH, et al. QRS prolongation in the prediction of clinical cardiac events in patients with acute heart failure: analysis of data from the Korean Acute Heart Failure Registry. Cardiology 2013;125:96–103.

27. Hong SJ, Oh J, Kang SM, et al. Clinical implication of right bundle branch block in hospitalized patients with acute heart failure: data from the Korean Heart Failure (KorHF) Registry. Int J Cardiol 2012;157:416–8.

28. Hamaguchi S, Tsuchihashi-Makaya M, Kinugawa S, et al. Anemia is an independent predictor of long-term adverse outcomes in patients hospitalized with heart failure in Japan - A report from the Japanese Cardiac Registry of Heart Failure in Cardiology (JCARE-CARD). Circ J 2009;73:1901–8.

29. Kajimoto K, Sato N, Takano T, on behalf of the investigators of the Acute Decompensated Heart Failure Syndrome (ATTEND) registry. Association between anemia, clinical features and outcome in patients hospitalized for acute heart failure syndromes. Eur Heart J Acute Cardiovasc Care 2015;29:1–11.

30. Hong N, Youn JC, Oh J, et al. Prognostic value of new-onset anemia as a marker of hemodilution in patients with acute decompensated heart failure and severe renal dysfunction. J Cardiol 2014;64:43–8.

31. Hunt SA, Abraham WT, Chin MH, et al. 2009 focused update incorporated into the ACC/AHA 2005 guidelines for the diagnosis and management of heart failure in adults: a report of the American College of Cardiology Foundation/American Heart Association Task Force on Practice Guidelines. J Am Coll Cardiol 2009;53:e1–90.

32. Youn YJ, Yoo B-S, Lee J-W, et al. Treatment performance measures affect clinical outcomes in patients with acute systolic heart failure-Report from the Korean Heart Failure Registry. Circ J 2012;76:1151–8.

33. Gheorghiade M, De Luca L, Fonarow GC, et al. Pathophysiologic targets in the early phase of acute heart failure syndromes. Am J Cardiol 2005;96(Suppl):11G–7G.

34. Testani JM, Chen J, McCauley BD, et al. Potential effects of aggressive decongestion during the treatment of decompensated heart failure on renal function and survival. Circulation 2010;122:265–72.

35. van der Meer P, Postmus D, Ponikowski P, et al. The predictive value of short-term changes in hemoglobin concentration in patients presenting with acute decompensated heart failure. J Am Coll Cardiol 2013;61:1973–81.

36. Oh J, Kang SM, Hong N, et al. Hemoconcentration is a good prognostic predictor for clinical outcomes in acute heart failure: data from the Korean Heart Failure (KorHF) Registry. Int J Cardiol 2013;168:4739–43.

37. Park JJ, Choi DJ, Yoon CH, et al. Prognostic value of C-reactive protein as an inflammatory and

N-terminal probrain natriuretic peptide as a neuro-humoral marker in acute heart failure (from the Korean Heart Failure Registry). Am J Cardiol 2014; 113:511–7.

38. Pascual-Figal DA, Bonaque JC, Redondo B, et al. Red blood cell distribution width predicts long-term outcome regardless of anemia status in acute heart failure patients. Eur J Heart Fail 2009;11:840–6.

39. Oh J, Kang SM, Won H, et al. Prognostic value of change in red cell distribution width 1 month after discharge in acute decompensated heart failure patients. Circ J 2012;76:109–16.

Biomarkers for Heart Failure in Asia

Arthur Mark Richards, MBChB, MD, PhD, DSc, FRCP, FRACP, FRSNZ[a],[b],*

KEYWORDS

- Heart failure • Biomarkers • Asia

KEY POINTS

- Contributions from the Asian biomedical community to the accumulating knowledge of biomarkers in heart failure have grown rapidly since 2000, with Japan's long-standing preeminence now facing the challenge of exponential growth in reports from China.
- A significant quantum of contributions also comes from Taiwan and South Korea, with a smaller number of high-quality reports from Singapore and Hong Kong.
- Since the 1980s Japan has made world-leading contributions in the discovery and application of the cardiac natriuretic peptides as biomarkers in heart failure.
- Leading centers in Asia have established rigorously designed and well-annotated clinical cohorts providing powerful platforms for the discovery and validation of biomarkers in heart failure.
- In the twenty-first century, Asian enquiry into biomarkers in heart failure covers the full gamut of circulating candidates, including peptides, cytokines, metabolites, nucleic acids, and other analytes.

INTRODUCTION

Asia is the most populous continent and it now harbors the greatest number of patients with heart failure (HF). World Health Organization figures indicate that China, India, Japan, and southeast Asia are home to an estimated 4.2 million, 1.3 to 4.6 million, 1 million, and 9 million people with HF respectively (totaling ~15.5–19.1 million). In comparison, case numbers are approximately 6 million in the United States and 15 million in Europe.

This article gives an overview of Asian contributions to discovery and application of biomarkers in HF. A simple estimate of the relative proportional contribution from key nations is presented.

Japan's leadership in cardiac natriuretic peptides is outlined. Examples are provided of the growing portfolio of diverse original reports from Asia with respect to multiple classes of circulating biomarkers. The interaction of East and West in this pivotal and burgeoning field is briefly discussed.

KEY PLAYERS

To provide a crude and noncomprehensive but consistent indicator of relative regional activity, a simple database search on PubMed was conducted applying the term "HF AND biomarkers AND x" (where x is the name of one of the 50 nations considered to comprise Asia). An arbitrary

Disclosures: Professor A.M. Richards sits on advisory boards and receives speaker's honoraria/travel support and research grants for diagnostic companies that manufacture cardiac biomarker assay systems, including Roche Diagnostics, Alere, Critical Diagnostics, and Abbott.

[a] Cardiac Department, Cardiovascular Research Institute, National University Heart Centre Singapore, 1E Kent Ridge Road, NUHS Tower Block, Level 9, Singapore 119228, Singapore; [b] Department of Medicine, Christchurch Hospital, Christchurch Heart Institute, University of Otago, PO Box 4345, Riccarton Avenue, Christchurch 8014, New Zealand

* Cardiac Department, Cardiovascular Research Institute, National University Heart Centre Singapore, 1E Kent Ridge Road, NUHS Tower Block, Level 9, Singapore 119228, Singapore

E-mail addresses: mdcarthu@nus.edu.sg; mark.richards@cdhb.health.nz

Heart Failure Clin 11 (2015) 551–561
http://dx.doi.org/10.1016/j.hfc.2015.07.007

decision was made to exclude Israel, Turkey, Cyprus, Georgia, and Russia from the search. These 5 countries (or parts thereof) are formally included in Asia but, from historical and/or cultural perspectives, are not commonly or universally perceived as Asian. Contributions from Hong Kong, which have a notable history, have been considered separately from China overall. Outputs were filtered to leave only those publications that (1) were dated from the year 2000 onwards, (2) were original (ie, reviews were excluded), (3) were peer reviewed, (4) were written in English, (5) applied to human rather than preclinical data or models, and (6) addressed candidate circulating biomarkers with potential utility in prediction of, diagnosis of, or risk stratification in human HF. **Table 1** gives the outcome of this search approach. Japan dominates with half (53%) of reports, followed by China with more than a quarter (29%). Taiwan (7.1%) and South Korea (3.4%) are strong contributors, with each of India, Iran, Oman, Pakistan, Singapore, Syria, Thailand, Vietnam, Hong Kong, and Saudi Arabia providing 0.1% to 1.8% of total Asian reports. The search yielded nil reports from the 32 other Asian nations.

The number of reports over time was examined for the 2 major contributing nations. The

proportion of reports from Japan over the 3 time periods 2000 to 2005, 2006 to 2010, and 2011 to 2015 decreased from 69% to 51% to 36% respectively, whereas the figures for China are 4%, 15%, and 33% respectively.

JAPAN AND THE NATRIURETIC PEPTIDE STORY

The best-established biomarkers in HF are the cardiac natriuretic peptides. Since their discovery in the 1980s they have filled what hitherto might be described as a marker vacuum and have become established clinical tools assisting in the diagnosis, risk stratification, and monitoring of acute and chronic HF. These applications, particularly for B-type natriuretic peptide (BNP) and N-terminal pro-BNP (NT-proBNP), are now endorsed in all major internationally acknowledged guidelines on the diagnosis and management of HF.[1,2] The contributions of Japanese workers to this field have been salutary. After the seminal report by de Bold and colleagues[3] proving the existence of an atrial natriuretic factor, Japanese investigators discovered the amino acid sequence of atrial natriuretic peptide (ANP), opening the way to its immunoassay and the elucidation of its biology.[3,4] In terms of therapeutic application of ANP, the Japanese experience is unique in using human recombinant ANP as a treatment to preserve cardiac ventricular function in the setting of acute myocardial infarction.[5] In 1988, Sudoh and colleagues[6] isolated the second member of the natriuretic peptide (NP) family from porcine brain. Brain NP was soon recognized to be a predominantly cardiac product and workers in Japan and elsewhere soon revealed the potential of plasma BNP as an index of cardiac health.[7] Data from Mukoyama and colleagues[8] clarified the atrial and ventricular contributions to synthesis and secretion of ANP and BNP. Increasing in parallel with increasing intracardiac pressures and with increasing clinical severity of HF, plasma BNP has come to be widely accepted as an excellent surrogate marker to assess baseline state and change in cardiac status. It is used in this way to (1) assist in the diagnosis of acute HF, (2) as a tool for titration of therapy and monitoring of compensated status, (3) for patient selection to therapeutic trials, as well as providing (4) a surrogate end point for such trials.[1,2,9]

The third member of the NP family, C-type NP (CNP) was also a Japanese discovery with initial isolation from porcine brain by Sudoh and colleagues[10] in 1990. A ubiquitous endothelium-based peptide, CNP is a paracrine growth factor[11] widely expressed in tissues including

Table 1
Published peer-reviewed original articles from Asian nations (2000–2015)

Nation	n	%
Japan	182	53
China	99	29
Taiwan	25	7.3
South Korea	12	3.5
India	3	0.9
Iran	3	0.9
Oman	1	0.3
Pakistan	4	1.2
Singapore	3	0.9
Syria	1	0.3
Thailand	3	0.9
Vietnam	1	0.3
Hong Kong	6	1.8
Saudi Arabia	1	0.3

As per PubMed search for "heart failure AND biomarkers in x", where x is the individual Asian nation. Further filtering included restriction to English publications, addressing circulating markers in clinical human HF designed to assess predictive, diagnostic, and/or prognostic performance of putative blood-borne markers. Thirty-two Asian nations had a zero return on this selective search.

the vascular endothelium.[12] In contrast with other cardiac natriuretic peptides (atrial NP, ANP, and BNP), and in keeping with the paracrine role of CNP, circulating concentrations of CNP are very low (<1 pM in healthy adults) so evaluating the role of CNP in the vasculature in humans is technically challenging. However, a coproduct (amino terminal proCNP [NT-proCNP]) of CNP gene expression is readily measured in plasma.[13] Values increase progressively in middle age, are higher in men, and are positively associated with hypertension and vascular risk factors.[14] Recently the potential biomarker function of circulating CNP and/or NT-proCNP has been explored in human HF.[15]

A recent Japanese-Western consensus on biomarkers reflected Japan's standing. The bulk of the report generated from this meeting and published in 2011 focuses on the cardiac NPs and East-West consensus statements were heavily underpinned by references to seminal publications from Japan between 1989 and 2010.[16] These publications documented leading Japanese contributions to discovery of the NPs, understanding of their production and processing, elucidation of their behavior in cardiovascular diseases, and their prognostic significance after myocardial infarction and in HF.[17–19]

THE HONG KONG HERITAGE IN BIOMARKERS FOR HEART FAILURE

Since the 1990s, Hong Kong investigators led by Professors John Sanderson and CM Yu, based in the Department of Medicine, Chinese University of Hong Kong, Prince of Wales Hospital, have produced a steady stream of original reports addressing circulating biomarkers in HF. They have often worked in concert with other centers of excellence with biomarker expertise, including the pioneering University of Otago Cardioendocrine Laboratory in Christchurch, New Zealand. Over a 20-year period their reports have elucidated the relationship of cardiac NPs (ANP and BNP) and nitric oxide to measures of diastolic dysfunction; confirmed the relationship of increasing plasma BNP to mortality in acute decompensated heart failure (ADHF); confirmed the increased levels of a range of other biomarkers in HF, including adrenomedullin; assessed the neurohormonal response to introduction of β-blocker therapy in HF; documented the correspondence between changes in plasma NT-proBNP and response to cardiac resynchronization therapy; and more recently this group reported the prognostic significance of serum albumin in HF with preserved ejection fraction (HFPEF).[20–26]

NEW DEVELOPMENTS FROM ASIA IN BIOMARKERS FOR HEART FAILURE

Original work on HF biomarkers in Asia currently covers the full gamut from affirmation of the diagnostic and prognostic performance of the known markers, previously assessed and developed in the West, to discovery of new candidates reflecting any of the varied aspects of the multifacetted pathophysiology of HF. Known circulating markers (with examples given here in parentheses) may report on myocardial mechanical strain (the NPs), systemic and renal neurohormonal activation (most importantly the renin-angiotensin-aldosterone system and sympathetic nervous system activation with corresponding increases in levels of plasma renin, angiotensin 2, aldosterone, and catecholamines), inflammation (C-reactive protein [CRP], interleukin [IL]-1, IL-6, tumor necrosis factor [TNF] alpha), renal challenge (creatinine, blood urea nitrogen [BUN], cystatin C), cardiac matrix derangement and fibrosis (procollagens, matrix metalloproteinases, and tissue inhibitors of metalloproteinase), and free radical status (assorted reactive oxygen species, myeloperoxidase). In addition to this classic array of known markers a burgeoning panoply of newcomer candidates have been the subject of multiple reports from around the globe, including Asia, in recent years. These candidates include more recently discovered cytokines such as growth differentiation factor 15 (GDF15). In the wake of increasing capacity in high-throughput omics technologies, new candidate markers are also being discovered among circulating nucleic acids and metabolomic profiles. **Box 1** lists candidate biomarkers addressed in reports from Asian centers since 2000.

Selected examples of current Asian initiatives in HF biomarkers are summarized here.

Peptide Biomarkers for Heart Failure in Asia

Singapore has recently accelerated its cardiovascular research effort. Initiatives in HF include a biomarker discovery effort spearheaded by the Cardiovascular Research Institute of the National University of Singapore. Workers at this center coordinate a nationwide HF cohort (Singapore Heart Failure Outcomes and Phenotypes [SHOP]). SHOP recruits patients at the time of admission for an episode of ADHF. Careful annotation and follow-up include serial echocardiographic imaging (soon to be supplemented with a large cardiac MRI substudy), serial blood sampling for biomarker discovery and evaluation, and clinical follow-up for clinical outcomes.[27] SHOP recently provided a pilot report examining concurrent plasma concentrations of key peptide/protein

Box 1
HF biomarkers included in publications from Asian investigators from 2000 to 2015: categorized according to physiologic role

Neurohormonal markers
- Cardiac NPs
  - BNPs (BNP1–BNP32, NT-proBNP1–NT-proBNP76, pro-BNP)
  - ANP, N-terminal proANP, midregion pro-ANP
- Renin-angiotensin-aldosterone system
  - Plasma renin activity
  - Angiotensin II
  - Aldosterone
- Adrenergic nervous system
  - Norepinephrine
  - Epinephrine
  - Dopamine
- Arginine vasopressin
  - Arginine vasopressin, copeptin
- Endothelial-derived peptides
  - Endothelin 1, big endothelin
  - Adrenomedullin

Renal markers
- BUN
- Cystatin C

Inflammatory markers
- C-reactive protein
- TNF-alpha
- Fas (APO-1)
- IL-1, IL-6, and IL-18

Advanced glycation endproducts/oxidative stress markers
- Pentosidine

Interstitial matrix remodeling markers
- Matrix metalloproteinases
- Tissue inhibitors of metalloproteinases
- Propeptide procollagen I, procollagen III

Myocyte injury markers
- Myosin light-chain kinase I
- Heart fatty acid binding protein
- Creatine kinase, creatine kinase MB fraction

Other/new markers
- ST2
- Growth differentiation factor 15
- Osteoprotegerin
- Adiponectin
- Galectin 3
- Coenzyme Q10

Metabolites
- Multiple amino acids, phosphatidylcholine moieties and so forth

Nonpeptide markers
- Serum albumin, urine albumin
- Hemoglobin, hemoglobin A1c
- Red cell distribution width

markers in patients with both HF with reduced ejection fraction (HFREF) and in HFPEF. NT-proBNP, GDF15, ST2, and high sensitivity troponin T (hsTnT) were all measured in SHOP and control non-HF cases in the first such concurrent multi-marker comparison of these 4 markers.[28] Clear increases in levels of GDF15 in HFPEF matched those observed in HFREF, whereas increased levels of NT-proBNP were muted despite similar ventricular filling pressures (E/e') in both HF phenotypes. The investigators suggested that inflammatory drivers may be more important than mechanical overload in the pathophysiology of HFPEF compared with HFPEF. A larger SHOP cohort has confirmed the prognostic power of plasma GDF15 in an Asian HF cohort. Further peptide combinations will be assessed in SHOP in data sets incorporating more than 1000 patients.

Reports from Asian centers have repeatedly confirmed the performance of BNP and NT-proBNP as prognostic markers in patients with acute and chronic HF. In many of these reports other candidate markers have been concurrently assessed and compared with the B-type cardiac peptides. Early in the century Tsutamoto and colleagues[29] measured circulating soluble fas (sFas), TNF-alpha, ANP, BNP, norepinephrine, and endothelin 1 in approximately 100 cases of ADHF followed for 3 years and ascertained sFas to be independently associated with measures of clinical severity of HF and independently predictive of outcomes; findings that are consistent with a significant role for immune activation and/or apoptosis in HF. Park and colleagues[30] studied 1608 patients with ADHF enrolled in the Korean registry. Over 12 months this cohort incurred 213 deaths independently predicted by both high sensitivity C reactive protein (hs-CRP) and NT-proBNP. Ho and colleagues[31] assessed combined markers of cardiomyocyte injury (cardiac troponin), inflammation (hs-CRP), and hemodynamic load (NT-proBNP) together with echocardiographic measures in predicting major adverse cardiac events in a small group of 87 patients with ADHF. The 2 markers with sustained prognostic power on multivariate analysis were NT-proBNP and E/e'; findings that are consistent with those from earlier Western studies. In the more chronic setting, Li and colleagues[32] assessed the prognostic performance of hs-CRP and big endothelin compared with NT-proBNP in more than 600 cases with dilated cardiomyopathy (DCM) seen at China's Fuwai hospital between 2005 and 2010. This study confirmed hs-CRP and NT-proBNP (but not big endothelin) as independent predictors of all-cause mortality. Izumiya and colleagues[33] confirmed the prognostic performance of GDF15 (along with BNP, age, and presence of atrial fibrillation) as independently prognostic in ~150 cases with HFREF.

In non-HF populations with coronary disease many markers (initially assessed in the setting of frank HF) have also been found to be predictive of later adverse events, including death or HF. Suzuki and colleagues[34] confirmed earlier reports of the predictive power of BNP after acute myocardial infarction. In 145 patients, plasma BNP measured at 3 to 4 months post-MI independently predicted death (n = 23) over 5-year follow-up, whereas univariate predictors including left ventricular ejection fraction and a previous history of HF did not. Kawagoe and colleagues[35] reported that transcardiac net uptake versus net production of adiponectin was associated with adverse events in coronary artery disease (CAD), including risk of subsequent HF. Chen and colleagues[36] contributed original information in their report on phospholipid transfer protein (PLTP), a modulator of lipoprotein metabolism and a participant in inflammatory processes and oxidative stress. Increasing PLTP level was associated with progressively impaired left ventricular (LV) systolic function in a well-characterized cohort (n = 495) with CAD.

Some efforts have been made to assess the possible utility of markers in detection of occult LV dysfunction or other cardiac abnormality in the ambulant community-based population. Nakamura and colleagues[37] reported that a plasma BNP level of 50 pg/mL in ~1000 well participants in a health screening study (in Iwate, Japan) had 90% sensitivity and 96% specificity, with an area under the receiver operating characteristic (ROC) curve of 0.97 in detecting an array of cardiac lesions in 39 subjects, including cases of lone atrial fibrillation/flutter, residual post-MI LV wall motion impairment (7 cases), hypertensive heart disease, and dilated cardiomyopathy.

News on Nonpeptide Markers from Asia

Nonpeptide markers, including BUN, plasma albumin, urinary albumin, hemoglobin, hemoglobin A1c, and red cell distribution width (RDW), have all been assessed in at-risk or frank HF cohorts (between 100 and 2500 in size) in Asian centers, and have been reported to be associated with adverse outcomes.[38–43]

Pentosidine, derived from ribose, is a marker of accumulated advanced glycation endproducts. Koyama and colleagues[44] delivered the first report evaluating associations between plasma pentosidine and both the diagnosis of HF and prognosis in HF. Plasma pentosidine, along with BNP, independently predicted adverse outcomes in HF.

A recent contribution from Taiwan identified metabolic signals in plasma associated with diagnosis and outcomes in HF. This article signals the arrival of metabolomics in the study of circulating biomarkers in HF. In both discovery and validation experiments in 515 patients with HF and appropriately matched controls, Chen and colleagues[36] provided panels of metabolites with similar diagnostic and superior prognostic abilities compared with BNP. A panel of circulating amino acids (histidine, phenylalanine, spermidine), together with phosphatidylcholine C34:4, discriminated between HF and control with a similar area under the curve (AUC) to BNP (**Fig. 1**). The ratio of asymmetric methyl arginine to arginine, butyrylcarnitine, and spermidine combined with the total of essential amino acids gave prognostic information on HF cases with superior prognostic performance to BNP (AUC, 0.85 vs 0.74). The derangement in metabolite profile was observed to shift toward control profiles as HF became well controlled, hinting at a potential role for serial measurement of metabolites in the titration of anti-HF therapy and monitoring of status in chronic HF.[45]

Nucleic Acids as Biomarkers in Heart Failure

MicroRNAs (miRNAs), a class of small noncoding RNAs, are increasingly recognized as playing key roles in cardiac differentiation and development, and in the cardiac response to stress and injury. Several miRNA arrays in human heart tissue have been reported and a few have addressed plasma miRNA profiles in HF. Tijsen and colleagues[46] suggested miR-423-5p as a diagnostic test in HF. The potential diagnostic utility for circulating microRNAs in HF or in distinguishing HFREF from HFPEF is unclear. Wong and colleagues from Singapore identified circulating microRNA profiles distinguishing both HFREF and HFPEF from non-HF controls and (for the first time) HFREF from HFPEF. MicroRNA profiling performed on whole blood and

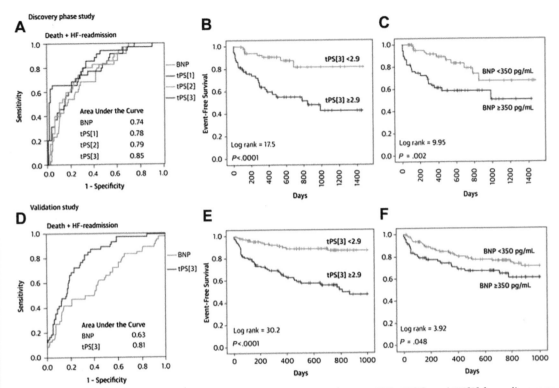

Fig. 1. (*A, D*) The ROC curves for comparing the prognostic values of BNP, tPS[1], tPS[2], and tPS[3] from discovery data; and BNP and tPS[3] in validation studies. (*B, C, E,* and *F*) The Kaplan-Meier curves of tPS[3] and BNP for predicting a composite event of all-cause death and HF-related rehospitalization in the discovery phase and the validation studies. tPS[1], tPS[2], tPS[3] are metabolite panels. (*From* Cheng ML, Wang CH, Shiao MS, et al. Metabolic disturbances identified in plasma are associated with outcomes in patients with heart failure diagnostic and prognostic value of metabolomics. J Am Coll Cardiol 2015;65(15):1517; with permission.)

corresponding plasma samples of controls and patients with HF identified 344 microRNAs differentially expressed among the 3 groups. In an independent cohort of controls, HFREF, and HFPEF, Wong and colleagues[47] validated 12 diagnostic microRNAs. Of these, miR-1233, miR-183-3p, miR-190a, miR-193b-3p, miR-193b-5p, miR-211-5p, miR-494, and miR-671-5p distinguished HF from controls. MiR-125a-5p, miR-183-3p, miR-193b-3p, miR-211-5p, miR-494, miR-638, and miR-671-5p were significantly expressed in HFREF, whereas miR-1233, miR-183-3p, miR-190a, miR-193b-3p, miR-193b- 5p, and miR-545-5p were significantly expressed in HFPEF compared with controls. Four microRNAs (miR-125a-5p, miR-190a, miR-550a-5p, and miR-638) showed differential expression between HFREF and HFPEF. Selective microRNA panels showed stronger discriminative power than NT-proBNP. Individual or multiple microRNAs used in combination with NT-proBNP increased discriminative performance, achieving perfect intergroup distinction. Pathway analysis revealed that the altered microRNA expressions were associated with several

mechanisms of potential significance in HF. Notably, Zhao and colleagues[48] reported 2 further plasma microRNAs (miR-210 and miR-30a) as distinguishing HF from control and confirming return of the levels of these 2 microRNAs to a fetal pattern in the presence of HF.

More data concerning the value of circulating microRNAs, in addition to circulating and long noncoding RNAs, as biomarkers in HF can be anticipated form Singapore, China, and elsewhere in Asia over coming years.

Genotyping for Heart Failure in Asia

Genetic variants can be considered to be forms of biomarkers. Few data exist on genetic variation related to HF in Asia. In the West, a large-scale genome-wide investigation of HF risk, the association of single-nucleotide polymorphisms with incident HF, was investigated by meta-analysis of data from 4 community-based prospective cohorts (the Atherosclerosis Risk in Communities Study, the Cardiovascular Health Study, the Framingham Heart Study, and the Rotterdam Study). Two loci were associated with incident HF and exceeded genome-wide significance: 15q22 (58.8 kb from USP3) among European-ancestry participants, and 12q14 (6.3 kb from LRIG3) among African-ancestry participants. The susceptibility loci were not shared between Europeans and Africans.[48,49] These genome-wide association studies support the hypothesis that common genetic variants, irrespective of specific proximate causal factors, contribute to risk of progression to overt HF. Findings are limited by interstudy heterogeneity and lack of uniform phenotyping. Notably, data from Asians are not yet available. The ASIAN-HF (Asian Sudden Cardiac Death in Heart Failure Registry) registry provides the opportunity for the largest HF genetic study yet undertaken and the first effort to discover genetic variants potentially directing the evolution to HFPEF versus HFREF phenotype in response to common cardiac challenges.[50]

The genotype best investigated for associations with risk and outcome of HF in Asia is the insertion/deletion polymorphism of the angiotensin-converting (ACE) gene. Insertion or deletion of an *ALU* repeat sequence of 287 base pairs in the kininase II (EC3.4.15.1; ie, ACE) gene results in II, ID, and DD genotypes with increased circulating ACE associated with the deletion state. Multiple reports from Western cohorts have associated the D allele with greater risk or worse outcomes in LV hypertrophy, ischemic heart disease, and DCM. Three reports between 1996 and 2004 indicate a low overall prevalence of the DD genotype in Han Chinese without difference in genotype distribution between controls and subjects with HF in either ischemic or idiopathic cardiomyopathy. It is possible that those occasional HF cases with the DD fare worse than those with ID or II genotypes.[51–53] Hong Kong workers have also investigated angiotensinogen (M235T) and angiotensin 2 type 1 receptor polymorphisms in HF in Chinese people. The increased prevalence of the M235T genotype in Chinese people was confirmed but no association with risk of, or outcomes in, HF were observed. The AC variant of the angiotensin receptor was linked to morbidity (hospital readmissions over 1-year follow-up) in univariate analyses but this association did not hold in multivariate analyses.[52]

Asia Is Organizing

The discovery and evaluation of clinically applicable biomarkers requires conduct of well-designed cohort studies in which rigorously standardized annotation of demographic and clinical characteristics is accompanied by scrupulous collection, processing, storage, and curating of biobanked blood and tissue samples. Asia is increasingly becoming organized in this respect with robust procedures and excellent cohorts under recruitment or established in Japan, Korea, Singapore, Taiwan, Hong Kong, and elsewhere. Examples include the Singapore SHOP cohort of more than 1000 patients with HF, as previously mentioned.[27] ASIAN-HF is a further Asia-wide HF registry led from Singapore with more than 50 contributing centers in 11 Asian countries aiming to recruit 8000 patients with HFREF and HFPEF (currently ~4600 patients) to address questions of clinical epidemiology and genetic variation in HF in Asia.[50] Other examples include the Japanese Cardiac Registry of Heart Failure in Cardiology (JCARE-CARD; >2000 patients), the Tohoku Heart Failure Registry (~500 patients), the CHART2 (Chronic Heart Failure Analysis and Registry in the Tohoku District 2) study (>2000 patients), the Korean Heart Failure Registry, and the Iwate screening programme.[30,37,38,40,41] Increasingly sophisticated laboratory technologies run by well-trained scientists are becoming coupled to well-run, fine-grained, registry-based data sets established or developing in an increasing number of Asian countries. The attention of both the diagnostics and pharmaceutical industries is increasingly turned toward Asia. The volume and quality of Asian contributions to biomarkers in HF is set to grow rapidly over the coming decade.

Markers When East Meets West

As data from Asia increase in both quality and quantum it has become increasingly clear that Western norms and HF phenotypes and their associations with circulating marker levels cannot necessarily be extrapolated to Asian populations. Patients with HF in Asia are, on average at first presentation, a decade younger than their Western counterparts. Examination of substrate causes suggests that diabetes and hypertension are more prominent causal factors in Asia than in the West. Comparisons of normative ranges of both electrocardiographic intervals and the normal ranges of echocardiographic dimensions indicate that, even in health, East and West may differ. In the largest collaborative effort of its kind to date, the EchoNoRMAL (Echocardiographic Normal Ranges Meta-Analysis of the Left Heart) consortium gathered echocardiographic information on more than 50,000 participants (including some thousands of Asian subjects) from more than 40 studies. Interethnic comparisons indicated that LV size was largest in white subjects, smaller in east Asian subjects, and smallest in south Asian subjects, even after indexation for body size[54] (**Fig. 2**). In the East South North West Trial, Gaggin

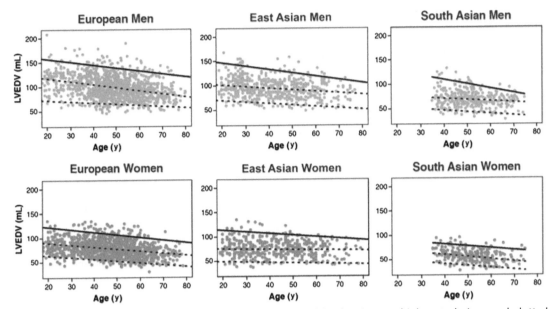

Fig. 2. Left ventricular end-diastolic volumes (LVEDV), measured by the Simpson biplane technique and plotted against age in years for 3 ethnicities: European (*left*), east Asian (*center*), and south Asian (*right*). (*From* Poppe KK. Ethnic-specific normative reference values for echocardiographic LA and LV size, LV mass, and systolic function: the EchoNoRMAL study. JACC Cardiovasc Imaging 2015;8(6):661; with permission.)

and colleagues[55] reported reference ranges for NT-proBNP and hsTnT in healthy age-matched and gender-matched populations of US (n = 565) and Vietnamese (592) subjects. Both the average concentration and percentage of the population with hsTnT levels greater than the limit of detection were significantly higher in the US participants. Similarly, mean NT-proBNP concentrations were more than 50% higher in normal US subjects than in Vietnamese healthy volunteers (*P*<.001). With increasing linkage between Asian and Western data sets, interethnic differences will be identified and defined over the next 10 years and, in association with this, differences in optimal interpretation of biomarker patterns in Asian compared with white populations will also be elucidated.

In summary, Asia has had an important presence in the study of biomarkers in HF from the 1980s onward. Japanese workers have been especially prominent and Japan remains the single largest Asian contributor. Internationally significant work has been done in Hong Kong from the 1990s and over the last decade China has become an increasingly major contributor. Asia is organizing its resources to couple rigorous collection of clinical material with excellent laboratory technology in several jurisdictions. Taiwan and Singapore are reporting an increasing number of original findings. Biomarker work in Asia is progressively moving beyond corroboration of findings in the West to initiatives in original discovery and evaluation of new candidate markers that may have particular application in Asian populations and phenotypes of disease, especially as clinicians further identify and define interethnic distinctions in normative values of markers and their ethnic-specific optimum interpretation in cardiovascular disease.

REFERENCES

1. Yancy CW, Jessup M, Bozkurt B, et al, American College of Cardiology Foundation; American Heart Association Task Force on Practice Guidelines. 2013 ACCF/AHA guideline for the management of heart failure: a report of the American College of Cardiology Foundation/American Heart Association Task Force on Practice Guidelines. J Am Coll Cardiol 2013;62:147–239.

2. McMurray JJ, Adamopoulos S, Anker SD, et al, ESC Committee for Practice Guidelines. Guidelines for the diagnosis and treatment of acute and chronic heart failure 2012: the Task Force for the Diagnosis and Treatment of Acute and Chronic Heart Failure 2012 of the European Society of Cardiology. Developed in collaboration with the Heart Failure Association (HFA) of the ESC. Eur Heart J 2012;33:1787–847.

3. de Bold AJ, Borenstein HB, Veress AT, et al. A rapid and potent natriuretic response to intravenous injection of atrial myocardial extract in rats. Life Sci 1981;28:89–94.

4. Oikawa S, Imai M, Ueno A, et al. Cloning and sequence analysis of cDNA encoding a precursor

for human atrial natriuretic polypeptide. Nature 1984;309:724–6.

5. Kuga H, Ogawa K, Oida A, et al. Administration of atrial natriuretic peptide attenuates reperfusion phenomena and preserves left ventricular regional wall motion after direct coronary angioplasty for acute myocardial infarction. Circ J 2003;67:443–8.

6. Sudoh T, Kangawa K, Minamino N, et al. A new natriuretic peptide in porcine brain. Nature 1988;332:78–81.

7. Nishikimi T, Kuwahara K, Nakagawa Y, et al. Complexity of molecular forms of B-type natriuretic peptide in heart failure. Heart 2013;99:677–9.

8. Mukoyama M, Nakao K, Hosoda K, et al. Brain natriuretic peptide as a novel cardiac peptide in humans. Evidence for an exquisite dual natriuretic peptide system, atrial natriuretic peptide and brain natriuretic peptide. J Clin Invest 1991;87:1402–12.

9. Troughton RW, Frampton CM, Brunner-La Rocca H-P, et al. Effect of B-type natriuretic peptide guided treatment of chronic heart failure on total mortality and hospitalization: an individual patient meta-analysis. Eur Heart J 2014;35:1559–67.

10. Sudoh T, Minamino N, Kangawa K, et al. C-type natriuretic peptide (CNP): a new member of natriuretic peptide family identified in porcine brain. Biochem Biophys Res Commun 1990;30(168):863–70.

11. Potter LR, Abbey-Hosch S, Dickey DM. Natriuretic peptides, their receptors, and cyclic guanosine monophosphate-dependent signaling functions. Endocr Rev 2006;27:47–72.

12. Sellitti DF, Koles N, Mendonça MC. Regulation of C-type natriuretic peptide expression. Peptides 2011; 32:1964–71.

13. Prickett TC, Yandle TG, Nicholls MG, et al. Identification of amino-terminal pro-C-type natriuretic peptide in human plasma. Biochem Biophys Res Commun 2001;286:513–7.

14. Prickett TC, Olney RC, Cameron VA, et al. Impact of age, phenotype and cardio-renal function on plasma C-type and B-type natriuretic peptide forms in an adult population. Clin Endocrinol 2013;78:783–9.

15. Lok DJ, Klip IT, Voors AA, et al. Prognostic value of N-terminal pro C-type natriuretic peptide in heart failure patients with preserved and reduced ejection fraction. Eur J Heart Fail 2014;16:958–66.

16. Maisel AS, Nakao K, Ponikowski P, et al. Japanese-Western consensus meeting on biomarkers. Int Heart J 2011;52:253–65.

17. Nishikimi T, Maeda N, Matsuoka H. The role of natriuretic peptides in cardiac protection. Cardiovasc Res 2006;69:318–28.

18. Yoshimura M, Yasue H, Okumura K, et al. Different secretion patterns of atrial natriuretic peptide and brain natriuretic peptide in patients with congestive heart failure. Circulation 1993;87:464–9.

19. Nishii M, Inomata T, Takehana H, et al. Prognostic utility of B-type natriuretic peptide assessment in stable low-risk outpatients with non-ischemic cardiomyopathy after decompensated heart failure. J Am Coll Cardiol 2008;51:2329–35.

20. Yu CM, Sanderson JE, Shum IO, et al. Diastolic dysfunction and natriuretic peptides in systolic heart failure. Higher ANP and BNP levels are associated with the restrictive filling pattern. Eur Heart J 1996; 17:1694–702.

21. Yu CM, Sanderson JE. Plasma brain natriuretic peptide–an independent predictor of cardiovascular mortality in acute heart failure. Eur J Heart Fail 1999;1:59–65.

22. Yu CM, Cheung BM, Leung R, et al. Increase in plasma adrenomedullin in patients with heart failure characterised by diastolic dysfunction. Heart 2001; 86:155–60.

23. Yu CM, Fung PC, Chan G, et al. Plasma nitric oxide level in heart failure secondary to left ventricular diastolic dysfunction. Am J Cardiol 2001;88: 867–70.

24. Fung JW, Yu CM, Yip G, et al. Effect of beta blockade (carvedilol or metoprolol) on activation of the renin-angiotensin-aldosterone system and natriuretic peptides in chronic heart failure. Am J Cardiol 2003;92:406–10.

25. Yu CM, Fung JW, Zhang Q, et al. Improvement of serum NT-ProBNP predicts improvement in cardiac function and favorable prognosis after cardiac resynchronization therapy for heart failure. J Card Fail 2005;11(5 Suppl):S42–6.

26. Liu M, Chan CP, Yan BP, et al. Albumin levels predict survival in patients with heart failure and preserved ejection fraction. Eur J Heart Fail 2012;14:39–44.

27. Santhanakrishnan R, Ng TP, Cameron VA, et al. The Singapore Heart Failure Outcomes and Phenotypes (SHOP) study and Prospective Evaluation of Outcome in Patients with Heart Failure with Preserved Left Ventricular Ejection Fraction (PEOPLE) study: rationale and design. J Card Fail 2013;19: 156–62.

28. Santhanakrishnan R, Chong JPC, Ng TP, et al. Growth differentiation factor 15, ST2, high sensitivity troponin T and N-terminal pro-B-type natriuretic peptide in heart failure with preserved versus reduced ejection fraction. Eur J Heart Fail 2012;14: 1338–47.

29. Tsutamoto T, Wada A, Maeda K, et al. Relationship between plasma levels of cardiac natriuretic peptides and soluble Fas: plasma soluble Fas as a prognostic predictor in patients with congestive heart failure. J Card Fail 2001;7:322–8.

30. Park JJ, Choi D-J, Yoon C-H, et al, on behalf of the KorHF Registry. Prognostic value of C-reactive protein as an inflammatory and N-terminal probrain natriuretic peptide as a neurohumoral marker in acute heart failure (from the Korean Heart Failure Registry). Am J Cardiol 2014;113:511–7.

31. Ho S-J, Feng A-N, Lee L-N, et al. Predictive value of predischarge spectral tissue Doppler echocardiography and N-terminal Pro-B-type natriuretic peptide in patients hospitalized with acute heart failure. Echocardiography 2011;28:303–10.

32. Li X, Chen C, Gan F, et al. Plasma NT pro-BNP, hs-CRP and big-ET levels at admission as prognostic markers of survival in hospitalized patients with dilated cardiomyopathy: a single-center cohort study. BMC Cardiovasc Disord 2014;14:67. Available at: http://www.biomedcentral.com/1471-2261/14/67.

33. Izumiya Y, Hanatani S, Kimura Y, et al. Growth differentiation factor-15 is a useful prognostic marker in patients with heart failure with preserved ejection fraction. Can J Cardiol 2014;30:338–44.

34. Suzuki S, Yoshimura M, Nakayama M, et al. Plasma level of B-type natriuretic peptide as a prognostic marker after acute myocardial infarction a long-term follow-up analysis. Circulation 2004;110: 1387–91.

35. Kawagoe J, Ishikawa T, Iwakiri H, et al. Association between adiponectin production in coronary circulation and future cardiovascular events in patients with coronary artery disease. Int Heart J 2014;55: 239–43.

36. Chen X, Sun A, Zou Y, et al. High PLTP activity is associated with depressed left ventricular systolic function. Atherosclerosis 2013;228:438–42.

37. Nakamura M, Endo H, Nasu M, et al. Value of plasma B type natriuretic peptide measurement for heart disease screening in a Japanese population. Heart 2002;87:131–5.

38. Miura M, Sakata Y, Nochioka K, et al. Prognostic impact of blood urea nitrogen changes during hospitalization in patients with acute heart failure syndrome. Circ J 2013;77:1221–8.

39. Uchikawa T, Shimano M, Inden Y, et al. Serum albumin levels predict clinical outcomes in chronic kidney disease (CKD) patients undergoing cardiac resynchronization therapy. Intern Med 2014;53: 555–61.

40. Takahashi J, Kohno H, Shimokawa H, on behalf of the CHART-2 Investigators. Urinary albumin excretion in heart failure with preserved ejection fraction: an interim analysis of the CHART 2 study. Eur J Heart Fail 2012;14:367–76.

41. Hamaguchi S, Tsuchihashi-Makaya S, Kinugawa S, et al, for the JCARE-CARD Investigators. Anemia is an independent predictor of long-term adverse outcomes in patients hospitalized with heart failure in Japan: a report from the Japanese Cardiac Registry of Heart Failure in Cardiology (JCARE-CARD). Circ J 2009;73: 1901–8.

42. Kishimoto I, Makino H, Ohata Y, et al. Hemoglobin A1c predicts heart failure hospitalization independent of baseline cardiac function or B-type natriuretic peptide level. Diabetes Res Clin Pract 2014;104:257–65.

43. He W, Jia J, Chen J, et al. Comparison of prognostic value of red cell distribution width and NT-proBNP for short-term clinical outcomes in acute heart failure patients. Int Heart J 2014;55:58–64.

44. Koyama Y, Takeishi Y, Arimoto T, et al. High serum level of pentosidine, an advanced glycation end product (AGE), is a risk factor of patients with heart failure. J Card Fail 2007;13: 199–206.

45. Cheng M-L, Wang C-H, Shiao M-S, et al. Metabolic disturbances identified in plasma are associated with outcomes in patients with heart failure diagnostic and prognostic value of etabolomics. J Am Coll Cardiol 2015;65:1509–20.

46. Tijsen AJ, Creemers EE, Moerland PD, et al. MiR423-5p as a circulating biomarker for heart failure. Circ Res 2010;106:1035–9.

47. Wong LL, Armugam A, Sepramaniam S, et al. Circulating microRNAs in heart failure with reduced and preserved left ventricular ejection fraction. Eur J Heart Fail 2015;17:393–404.

48. Smith NL, Felix JF, Morrison AC, et al. Association of genome-wide variation with the risk of incident heart failure in adults of European and African ancestry: a prospective meta-analysis from the Cohorts for Heart and Aging Research in Genomic Epidemiology (CHARGE) Consortium. Circ Cardiovasc Genet 2010;3:256–66.

49. Morrison AC, Felix JF, Cupples LA, et al. Genomic variation associated with mortality among adults of European and African ancestry with heart failure: the Cohorts for Heart and Aging Research in Genomic Epidemiology Consortium. Circ Cardiovasc Genet 2010;3:248–55.

50. Lam CS, Anand I, Zhang S, et al. Asian Sudden Cardiac Death in Heart Failure (ASIAN-HF) registry. Eur J Heart Fail 2013;15:928–36.

51. Huanga W, Xieb C, Zhoua H, et al. Association of the angiotensin-converting enzyme gene polymorphism with chronic heart failure in Chinese Han patients. Eur J Heart Fail 2004;6:23–7.

52. Sanderson JE, Young RP, Yu CM, et al. Lack of association between insertion/deletion polymorphism of the angiotensin-converting enzyme gene and end-stage heart failure due to ischemic or idiopathic dilated cardiomyopathy in the Chinese. Am J Cardiol 1996;77:1008–10.

53. Sanderson JE, Yu CM, Young RP, et al. Influence of gene polymorphisms of the renin-angiotensin system on clinical outcome in heart failure among the Chinese. Am Heart J 1999;137:653–7.

54. EchoNoRMAL (Echocardiographic Normal Ranges Meta-Analysis of the Left Heart) Collaboration, EchoNoRMAL Echocardiographic Normal Ranges

Meta-Analysis of the Left Heart Collaboration. Ethnic-specific normative reference values for echocardiographic LA and LV size, LV mass, and systolic function: the EchoNoRMAL Study. JACC Cardiovasc Imaging 2015;8:656–65.

55. Gaggin HK, Dang PV, Do LD, et al. Reference interval evaluation of high-sensitivity troponin T and N-terminal B-type natriuretic peptide in Vietnam and the US: the North South East West Trial. Clin Chem 2014;60:758–64.

Heart Transplant in Asia

Rungroj Krittayaphong, MD, FACC, FESC[a],*, Aekarach Ariyachaipanich, MD[b,c]

KEYWORDS

- Heart transplant • Asia • Heart failure

KEY POINTS

- In Asia the heart transplant program began in Taiwan and Thailand in 1987. At present, there are at least 10 Asian countries that have experience in heart transplant operations.
- Data from registries in each Asian country have shown a trend toward an increase in the number of heart transplants, mainly due to the implementation of legislation for organ donation.
- The underlying heart disease for heart transplant recipients was nonischemic cardiomyopathy followed by ischemic cardiomyopathy, similar to reports from Western countries. However, valvular heart disease was more common in Asia.
- Survival at 1, 5, and 10 years after heart transplant in Asia was similar to that in Western countries.

INTRODUCTION

The history of heart transplant began with Alexis Carrel who conducted experiments on heterotopic heart transplant in animals.[1] For this work, he received the Nobel Prize in medicine and physiology in 1912. It took a long time before the first successful attempt in humans on 3 December, 1967, by Christiaan Bernard at the Groote Schuur Hospital in South Africa.[2] Since then, heart transplant has become the treatment of choice for helping selected patients with end-stage heart disease. There have been tremendous advances in the field, such as donor and recipient selection, immunosuppression management, and prevention of complications. The number of heart transplants has been growing. Annually, more than 4100 new heart transplants were reported to the International Society of Heart and Lung Transplantation (ISHLT) registry from worldwide. Data from North America and Europe make up around 90% of this data set.[3] The ISHLT estimates that there are 33% of heart transplant activities that are not submitted to the global registry. This makes the

registry unlikely to mirror the actual heart transplant activities, especially in Asia. Complete and updated data regarding heart transplant in Asia are unavailable. Countries that participate in the ISHLT registry include India, Iran, Israel, Japan, Korea, and Saudi Arabia.[4] With all these countries combined, there are only 10 heart transplant centers from Asia that participate in ISHLT registry (**Table 1**). This article reviews the history and current status of heart transplantation in Asia.

HEART FAILURE IN ASIA
Prevalence of Heart Failure

There are many differences between Western and Asian countries not only in ethnicity but also in income, population index, culture, health care system, lifestyle, and dietary pattern.[5–7]

Owing to the increase in the elderly population and a reduction in mortality of patients with myocardial infarction, the prevalence of heart failure has been reported to be increased both in the Western population[8] and in the Asian population.[9] The population living with heart failure has been

Conflict of interest: Nothing to declare for both authors.
[a] Division of Cardiology, Department of Medicine, Siriraj Hospital, Mahidol University, 2 Wanglang Road, Bangkoknoi, Bangkok 10700, Thailand; [b] Excellent Center for Organ Transplantation, King Chulalongkorn Memorial Hospital, Thai Red Cross Society, 1873 Rama 4 Road, Patumwan, Bangkok 10330, Thailand; [c] Division of Cardiology, Department of Medicine, Chulalongkorn University, 1873 Rama 4 Road, Patumwan, Bangkok 10330, Thailand
* Corresponding author.
E-mail address: rungroj.kri@mahidol.ac.th

Table 1
The list of countries in Asia and number of heart transplant centers that participate in the ISHLT registry

Country	Number of Centers
India	1
Iran	2
Israel	2
Japan	2
The Republic of Korea	2
Saudi Arabia	1

estimated to be approximately 1.9% in the United States, whereas the number is 1% in Japan and 1.3% in China.[10] Overall, the prevalence of heart failure in Asia is 1.26% to 6.7%.[6] Heart failure as the primary diagnosis of hospital admission accounts for 1,179,151 admissions in the United States in 2010 or 3.04% of total hospital admissions compared with 174,957 admissions in Japan or 1.24% of total admissions and 57,147 admissions in Korea or 0.78% of total admissions.[10]

Patients' Characteristics of Heart Failure in Asia

There are some racial differences in the prevalence of heart disease, including coronary artery disease (CAD), which is more common in Western countries,[7] and valvular heart disease, such as rheumatic heart disease (RHD), which is more common in Eastern countries.[11] The cause of heart failure in China was mainly cardiomyopathy and RHD, except in the urban areas in China, such as Shanghai, where CAD is a more common cause.[12]

The main differences in heart failure between the Western and Asian populations are the age and the severity of heart failure at presentation.[13,14] An Asian population that was admitted with heart failure in the Acute Decompensated Heart Failure National Registry (ADHERE) was almost 10 years younger than the Western population. The younger age of presentation in Asian countries would suggest that the burden from heart failure and its economic impact should be more than in Western countries. Heart failure in Asian populations tend to have more dyspnea, dyspnea at rest, rales, low blood pressure, and more use of intravenous inotropes and mechanical ventilation when compared with Western populations.[14] From the ADHERE registry, the proportion of patients with Heart failure with reduced ejection fraction (HFREF) and Heart failure with preserved ejection fraction (HFPEF) was similar between the Western population (50% HFREF)[15] and the Asia-Pacific population, of which 90% came from an Asian population (53% HFREF).[14]

Advanced Heart Failure in Asia

Heart failure functional class III–IV accounts for 27% to 30% of patients with heart failure in the United States.[16] The data from the heart failure registry in an Asian population showed that the proportion of patients in functional class III and IV in chronic heart failure was 21% in Shingen, Japan,[17] and 17% in the Chronic Heart Failure Analysis and Registry in Tohoku district (CHART1) study.[18] Patients with advanced heart failure despite optimal medication and device management should be referred to specialists in heart failure that needs multidisciplinary care. These patients should be considered candidates for mechanical circulatory supports (MCSs) or heart transplant.[10,16]

Heart Failure Management in Asia

Many standard medications that benefit the reduction of heart failure mortality and morbidity, such as angiotensin converting enzyme inhibitors, angiotensin receptor blockers, and β-blockers, are used at a significantly lower rate at hospital discharge compared with Western populations, especially the β-blockers (41% vs 74%).[14,19] Certain investigations such as the estimation of the levels of brain natriuretic peptide (BNP) or N-terminal proBNP and echocardiography were used to a lesser extent in the Asian population than in the Western population.[14]

Heart Failure Outcome in Asia

The mortality rate of heart failure has been improved in the past decade as a result of clinical trials that showed the benefit of medications that act on neurohormonal systems. The mortality during hospitalization and at 1 and 5 years were approximately 7%, 25% to 30%, and more than 50%, respectively.[13] The mortality data were not different between the Western and Asian populations.

HEART TRANSPLANT IN ASIA
History

As in various other regions in the world, heart transplantation has been established in Asia many decades ago. The first heart transplant in Asia was performed in 1968 by Dr Juro Wada at Sapporo Medical University, Japan.

Initial experiences were met with poor outcomes, until cyclosporine was used in 1980. The heart transplant era began again in Asia in 1987 at Taiwan[20] and Thailand.[21] The first survey of heart transplants in Asia was published in 1999.[22] This survey reported the heart transplant activity from 1987 to 1996. There were a total of 380 cases from 8 countries. During that reported period, heart transplant operations were performed in Taiwan (178 cases), Thailand (95 cases), Singapore (12 cases), South Korea (65 cases), Hong Kong (8 cases), China (7 cases), India (12 cases), and Philippines (3 cases). A follow-up survey in 2004 also captured the heart and lung transplantation activity.[23] At present, there are reports of heart transplant activity from other countries also, including Japan, Malaysia, Saudi Arabia, Iran, Bangladesh, and Vietnam.

Incidence and Prevalence

It is hard to estimate the actual current number of heart transplants in Asia. From survey, the total number of heart transplants in Asia during each 5-year period of 1991–1995, 1995–1999, and 1998–2002 were 247, 540, and 460, respectively.[23–25] **Table 2** summarizes transplant activities, recipient and donor demographics, and outcome of heart transplant in countries in Asia, including Hong Kong,[26,27] Iran,[28,29] Japan,[30,31] Korea,[32,33] Saudi Arabia,[34,35] Singapore,[36] Taiwan,[37,38] and Thailand[39] in comparison with data from ISHLT.[3] Information was extracted mainly from national-level published reports. In some countries, the largest series from that country was reviewed.

Half of the total heart transplants in Asia were done in Taiwan. In Taiwan, 1354 hearts transplants have been performed between 1987 and 2012, which makes it the most experienced country in this region. Taiwan is currently performing around 90 heart transplants each year.[38] Among other countries, the numbers of cases since the initiation of the program are as follows: Korea, 552; Saudi Arabia, 249; Japan, 133; Iran, 122; Thailand, 97; Hong Kong, 77; and Singapore, 40 (see **Table 2**). These numbers may not represent the actual volume because of lack of updated published reports from that country. **Fig. 1** shows the number of heart transplants in each Asian country by year.[26,28,31,32,34,36,37,40]

Recipient and Cause of End-Stage Heart Disease

Heart transplantation is not a suitable treatment for every patient. There is no region-wide regulatory organization to regulate candidate selection. The candidacy criteria and processes vary from country to country. In general, the candidate selection criteria were similar to those in the Western countries. For example, in Japan, criteria for candidates included a preferred age less than 60 years, functional class III or IV despite conventional treatment, life-threatening arrhythmia unresponsive to conventional treatment, and prolonged or repeated hospitalization due to heart failure. Patients were considered unsuitable if they had severe noncardiac disease, active peptic ulcer, active infection, severe diabetes mellitus, morbid obesity, drug or alcoholic abuse, human immunodeficiency virus infection, psychiatric disease, or pulmonary hypertension with pulmonary vascular resistance more than 6 Wood units unresponsive to vasodilators.[41]

Developed countries such as Taiwan, Hong Kong, Singapore, Korea, and Japan have an average recipient age of 49, 47, 45, 43, and 41 years, respectively, which is greater when compared with Iran, Saudi Arabia, and Thailand (average recipient age of 29, 35, and 35 years, respectively). Overall, the recipients in Asia were younger (unknown statistical significance) when compared with data from ISHLT registry (median recipient age of 54 years) (see **Table 2**). Regarding gender, recipients in Asia were more commonly male. The men to woman ratios were the same as in the ISHLT registry.

The causes for recipients to undergo heart transplant in most Asian countries were comparable with those of the global registry. CAD was the cause in 27% to 53% in most countries. According to ISHLT registry, CAD was diagnosed in 36% of patients. The CAD portions in Saudi Arabia, Iran, Japan, and Korea are smaller at 10%. With RHD still a common condition in Asia, valvular heart disease was the most common (32%) cause of end-stage heart failure in Hong Kong.[26]

Screening for Donors

Although donor selection criteria may be varied among different countries, the overall strategy was more or less similar. For example, the donor's criteria from the Korean Task Force of Organ Transplant were (1) not more than 45 years (men) or 50 years (women), (2) ABO compatibility, (3) no history of chest injury or cardiac surgery, (4) no sepsis, (5) no previous myocardial infarction by electrocardiography, (6) normal results on echocardiogram, and (7) body weight deviation not more than 20%.[32]

The estimated age of donor in Asia was 30 to 40 years, which is the same as in the Western population. Iran has the lowest mean age of donor at

Table 2
The transplant activities, recipient and donor demographics, and outcome of heart transplant in countries in Asia

Country[a]	ISHLT[b,3]	Hong Kong[26,27]	Iran[28,29]	Japan[30,31]	Korea[32,33]	Saudi Arabia[34,35]	Singapore[36]	Taiwan[37,38]	Thailand[39]
First transplant	1967	1992	1993	1999	1992	1989	1990	1987	1987
Reported period	2006–2013	1992–2006	1993–2006	1999–2013	1992–2011	1989–2013	1990–2007	1987–2012	1987–1997
Total transplants during reported period	26,294	77	122	185	552	249	40	1354	97
Estimated annual transplants	4196	7–12	18	13	98	21	4	80	10
Recipient									
Mean age (y)	54	47	29	38	43	35	45	49	35
Age range	24–67[c]	19–65	1.5–74	10–62	0–77	13–57	14–64	0.3–74	3–66
Male/female ratio	3.2:1	4:1	2.3:1	2.6:1	2.4:1	4:1	5.6:1	4:1	2.9:1
Underlying heart disease									
Nonischemic cardiomyopathy (%)	55	34	76	64	71	70	43	52	59
Ischemic cardiomyopathy (%)	36	14	10	8	11	13	53	33	31
Valvular heart disease	3	34	—	0	—	12	—	8	7
Others (%)	6	18	14	28	18	5	4	7	3
Preoperative inotropic support (%)	42	23	—	9	10	26	—	—	—
Preoperative MCS (%)	35	—	—	90	1	15	—	32	—
Donor age (y)	35	39	26	43	33	—	38	37.7	—
Survival (%)									
1 y	84	85	57	98	96	87	~80–90	81	~90
5 y	~75	80	40	93	87	~80	~75	68	70
10 y	~57[d]	—	—	90	74	—	~60	51	58 at 8th y

Data are extracted from available national-level published reports. Information from a large single-center experience from Iran, Saudi Arabia were added.
[a] Other Asian countries that have also performed heart transplant include Bangladesh, India, Malaysia, Philippines, China, and Vietnam. No comprehensive data available.
[b] Data from 2006 to June 2013 era.
[c] Median (5th–95th percentiles).
[d] Data from 2002 to 2005 era.

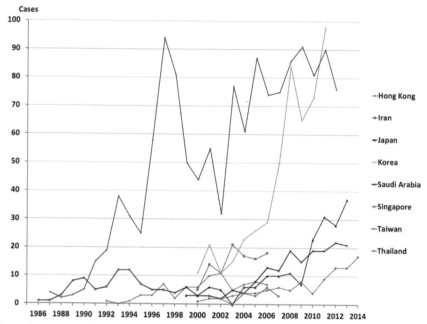

Fig. 1. Number of heart transplants in each Asian country by year.

25.9 years, and Japan has the oldest mean age of donor at 42.9 years (see **Table 2**).

For the operation, either atrial or bicaval anastomosis was performed, depending on centers' experiences. In the early 2000s, many centers mainly used the bicaval technique.

In Japan, because of the limited number of donors, special donor evaluation and management system has been developed. This system consisted of medical consultants who can evaluate and give intensive strategy to maximize suitable organs from the donor. By doing this, the number of organs per donor significantly increased.[31] Many heart donors required high-dose inotropes.

No heart transplant recipient had primary graft failure (PGF).

Survival

In the global registry data annually published by the ISHLT,[3] the survival rate was excellent, with a 1-year survival rate of 84% after cardiac transplant and with 50% of the patients surviving more than 10 years.

The heart transplant results in Asia reported a survival rate that was comparable with or slightly inferior to the results reported from the ISHLT registry (see **Table 2**). **Fig. 2** shows a survival graph

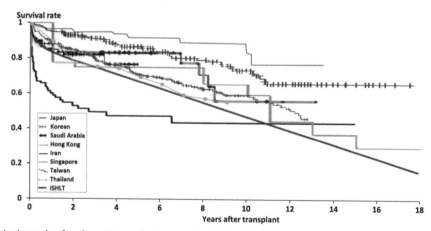

Fig. 2. Survival graph after heart transplant operation among Asian countries compared with data from ISHLT.

after heart transplant operation among Asian countries compared with data from ISHLT.[3,26,29,31,33,35,36,39,42]

Heart transplant results in Japan are exceptionally excellent compared with other countries in Asia or worldwide. A recent report from Japan revealed survival rates after heart transplant of 98% at 1 year, 93% at 5 years, and 90% at 10 years.[31] The results were achieved despite a smaller number of transplants per center, higher donor age, and more frequent use of MCS before transplantation (90% of recipients), when compared with the ISHLT registry.

HEART TRANSPLANT IN SPECIAL SITUATIONS
Rheumatic Heart Disease

A study of 23 patients with end-stage RHD and 226 patients with DCM from the Taiwan heart transplant program showed that the outcome of heart transplant in patients with end-stage RHD was not as good as that in patients with DCM.[43] The 15-year survival rate was 23% in the RHD group and 46% in the DCM group.

Elderly

An outcome comparison between a young and an elderly population after heart transplant from Korea showed that early mortality and rejection rate was not higher in the elderly population. Long-term survival was not different.[44]

Hepatitis B Virus Infection

About 8% of the 412 heart transplant recipients in Taiwan were positive for the hepatitis B antigen. Reactivation of hepatitis B virus (HBV) infection occurred in 68% of patients. All patients had a clinical response with lamivudine. Three recipients with negative HBV antigen received hearts from HBV-positive donors. All 3 patients were given HBV vaccination. Two of the 3 were not infected by HBV after heart transplant.[45]

POST–HEART TRANSPLANT CARE
Immunosuppression and Rejection

Literature reviews showed that centers in Asia used the same strategy as in Europe and North America to control and treat rejection. A 3-drug immunosuppressant regimen consisting of a calciurin inhibitor, myocophenolate, and a steroid was commonly used. The steroid was weaned down with the aim to stop at 6 to 12 months after transplant. In selected patients, the proliferation signal inhibitor (mammalian target of rapamycin inhibitor) is used instead or along with reduced doses of cyclosporine.

The absolute conclusion regarding the induction of an immunosuppression regimen is not available, but there are uses of polyclonal anti-lymphocyte globulin/anti-thymocyte globulin or interleukin-2 receptor antagonists reported.

Endomyocardial Biopsy

A Taiwan study of 411 patients who underwent heart transplant showed that rejection most commonly occurs within 2 years after transplant. Therefore, a scheduled biopsy should be routinely performed within 2 years. After 3 years, because the rejection rate is low, an event-driven biopsy may be preferred.[46]

HEART TRANSPLANT COMPLICATION
Primary Graft Failure

PGF is defined as impairment in systolic function of the graft usually occurring within 24 hours and requiring intravenous inotropic agents and had a poor outcome. A report from Taiwan showed the incidence of this condition to be 36%,[42] which is greater than in Western countries.[47] This difference may be from the difference in the definition of PGF. MCS devices, inotropes, and intensified immunosuppressants especially steroid pulse are commonly required. Retransplant is also a treatment option when available.

Cardiac Allograft Vasculopathy

Cardiac allograft vasculopathy (CAV) is common due to accelerated atherosclerosis of the transplant heart. It leads to cardiovascular complications and accounts for an increased risk of mortality. The prevalence of CAV diagnosed by angiography in a Western population was 11%, 22%, and 45% at 1, 2, and 4 years.[48] However, the prevalence was much less in an Asian population.[49] Prevention of accelerated atherosclerosis may improve long-term outcome as was shown in a previous Asian population study in which the use of statins was associated with better survival.[50]

Cardiac Arrhythmia

Prevalence of posttransplant cardiac arrhythmia was 31%.[51] Atrial tachyarrhythmia was more common than ventricular tachyarrhythmia or bradyarrhythmia. Sudden cardiac death rate was increased in patients with ventricular arrhythmia or more than 1 type of cardiac arrhythmia. Prevalence of atrial arrhythmia was similar to a previous report from the Western population.[52]

Malignancy

A previous report showed that malignancy is the cause of death in 335 patients who live longer than 5 years after heart transplant.[53] The cumulative incidence of malignancy reported from Taiwan was much less than from ISHLT. The incidence from ISHLT at 1, 5, and 10 years were 2.9%, 15.1%, and 31.9%, respectively, compared with 1%, 4.2%, and 8.1% in a Chinese population. Skin cancer was the type of malignancy that explains most of the difference.

The Asian population also has a trend toward an increased risk of non-Hodgkin lymphoma, bronchus, and trachea and lung cancers.[54]

Infection

Infection is common in patients after heart transplant because of treatment with immunosuppressive agents. Tuberculosis is more common in the Asian than in the Western population. Approximately 2.8% of posttransplant Taiwanese patients become infected with tuberculosis.[55]

Mechanical Circulatory Support Devices in Asia

The left ventricular assist device (LVAD) has been used successfully in Asian countries,[56] especially in countries that have a long heart transplant waiting list such as Japan.

Korean data from 2007 to 2012 showed that 35% were bridged with LVAD.[57] Median duration of the ventricular assist device was 227 days. In-hospital mortality was not different from those without bridging (5% vs 1%). Late survival was similar.

Barriers and Key to Success in Heart Transplant Program in Asia

Asia is the biggest continent on earth with many ethnic groups. Each center in Asia faced unique problems such as the culture barrier, absence of legal support, lack of technical experience, economic burden, and unsatisfactory organizational networks, which added on to other issues, such as limitation of a donor, that other parts of the world were facing. By acknowledging these limitations and learning from other countries in the same region, heart transplant activities can be improved.

Law

Having a legal framework to clarify brain death helps balancing transplant activities and the donor's rights which is the important step in improving transplant activities. For example, since 2010, the Japanese law on brain death and organ transplant has been revised to allow family to give consent for the donors. It resulted in a 10-fold increase in organ donation in Japan. This revision also allows children younger than 15 years to become a donor, leading to the first pediatric heart transplant from a pediatric donor in Japan.

Ethical Issue

One has to respect and understand beliefs and cultures in different populations. Misunderstanding may translate into failure to provide a life-saving treatment such as transplant. Traditionally, Muslims believe that body desecration in life or death is forbidden, and this may affect organ transplant. Many reports shed light on this area and clearly show that the Islamic faith supports organ donation and transplant to save lives. Similarly, some Buddhist families may believe that taking an organ from a brain-dead person prevents them from having a normal next life. One cannot overstate the importance of culture-sensitive issues in transplant.

Infrastructure

Besides the learning curve of a new clinical transplant skill, support from a centrally organized system for donor identification, management, and organ allocation is important for sustainable transplant activities in a country. During the last 10 years, the national-level organization for donor and organ management and allocation has been established in most countries in Asia.[25]

Donor Shortage

Shortage of organ donation has been a major problem worldwide. This seems to be a bigger problem in Asia than in Western countries.

Many Asian countries have a much longer waiting time than Western countries. The donation rate is lower in Asian countries than in Western countries. The donation rate per million population in Japan was only 0.08, compared with 7.3 and 5.3 in the United States and Spain, respectively. The mean waiting time in Korea was 552 days. In Japan, candidates were on the waiting list for more than 2 years before transplant. This long waiting time results in a higher death rate while waiting for suitable donor and higher rate of MCS. It is not uncommon for a patient to go from one country to another to undergo evaluation for heart transplant.[25]

Great efforts have to be implemented to solve these issues. Public education may play an important role. Intensive care doctors should inform the relatives after the victim has a declared brain death and the possibility to donate organs.

Limitation of Data

Because of significant publication bias and missing data, it is hard to discern the realistic view of the number and status of heart transplants in each Asian country. For example, the data from the People's Republic of China, which is believed to have the largest number of cadaveric organ transplants in Asia, is not available. In India, it is currently estimated that there are 100 heart transplants performed each year. However, these data are not available in the medical literature.

The act of data collection from each country is required to be discussed seriously. Collaborations within Asia are urgently needed to understand differences in race, culture, and outcome in transplant compared with Western countries. Fortunately, there are a few countries, such as Taiwan, Japan, Saudi Arabia, Korea, and Iran, that actively report and update their experiences and progress on heart transplant.

Even though it is less related to heart transplant, one cannot disregard the global concerns of unethical living unrelated organ donation, organ harvesting, and transplant tourism in Asia. Comprehensive, updated information regarding donors and recipients are likely to help clarify this view point and help transplant activities in Asia.

Future

One shall remember that it was in Asia that Dr Vladimir P. Demikhov, a legendary surgeon from Russia, pioneered in thoracic transplant and the use of an artificial heart more than half a century ago. Heart transplant has now become a widely available treatment option for end-stage heart failure. In Asia, each country is in various developmental stages. Clinical success may be different. The religious and social beliefs and legal structure may exert a great influence on patients. As the most populated region of the world, there is a need and expectation to explore and expand transplantation in this geographic area.

SUMMARY

The number of people living with advanced heart failure is increasing in Asia. Many of these patients are candidates for heart transplant. Data from registries and surveys showed that many countries in Asia currently perform heart transplant operation. There are many barriers in Asian countries such as law and belief. Each country has its own strategy to overcome these barriers. The number of heart transplants has been increasing during the last decade. The survival rate after heart transplant is similar to global data.

REFERENCES

1. DiBardino DJ. The history and development of cardiac transplantation. Tex Heart Inst J 1999;26:198–205.
2. Barnard CN. The operation. A human cardiac transplant: an interim report of a successful operation performed at Groote Schuur Hospital, Cape Town. S Afr Med J 1967;41:1271–4.
3. Lund LH, Edwards LB, Kucheryavaya AY, et al. The registry of the International Society for Heart and Lung Transplantation: thirty-first official adult heart transplant report–2014; focus theme: retransplantation. J Heart Lung Transplant 2014;33:996–1008.
4. ISHLT Registries 2014 Slides. Introduction/general statistics. The International Society for Heart and Lung Transplantation. 2015. Available at: http://www.ishlt.org/registries/slides.asp?slides=heartLung Registry. Accessed April 30, 2015.
5. Bi Y, Jiang Y, He J, et al. Status of cardiovascular health in Chinese adults. J Am Coll Cardiol 2015; 65:1013–25.
6. Sakata Y, Shimokawa H. Epidemiology of heart failure in Asia. Circ J 2013;77:2209–17.
7. Sasayama S. Heart disease in Asia. Circulation 2008;118:2669–71.
8. Heidenreich PA, Albert NM, Allen LA, et al. Forecasting the impact of heart failure in the United States: a policy statement from the American Heart Association. Circ Heart Fail 2013;6:606–19.
9. Jiang H, Ge J. Epidemiology and clinical management of cardiomyopathies and heart failure in China. Heart 2009;95:1727–31.
10. Ponikowski P, Anker SD, AlHabib KF, et al. Heart failure: preventing disease and death worldwide. ESC Heart Failure 2014;1:4–25.
11. Marijon E, Mirabel M, Celermajer DS, et al. Rheumatic heart disease. Lancet 2012;379:953–64.
12. Lee S, Khurana R, Gerard Leong KT. Heart failure in Asia: the present reality and future challenges. Eur Heart J Suppl 2012;14(Suppl A):A51–5.
13. Adams KF Jr, Fonarow GC, Emerman CL, et al. Characteristics and outcomes of patients hospitalized for heart failure in the United States: rationale, design, and preliminary observations from the first 100,000 cases in the Acute Decompensated Heart Failure National Registry (ADHERE). Am Heart J 2005;149:209–16.
14. Atherton JJ, Hayward CS, Wan Ahmad WA, et al. Patient characteristics from a regional multicenter database of acute decompensated heart failure in Asia Pacific (ADHERE International-Asia Pacific). J Card Fail 2012;18:82–8.
15. West R, Liang L, Fonarow GC, et al. Characterization of heart failure patients with preserved ejection fraction: a comparison between ADHERE-US registry and ADHERE-International registry. Eur J Heart Fail 2011;13:945–52.

16. Miller LW, Guglin M. Patient selection for ventricular assist devices: a moving target. J Am Coll Cardiol 2013;61:1209–21.

17. Goda A, Yamashita T, Suzuki S, et al. Prevalence and prognosis of patients with heart failure in Tokyo: a prospective cohort of Shinken Database 2004–5. Int Heart J 2009;50:609–25.

18. Shiba N, Shimokawa H. Chronic heart failure in Japan: implications of the CHART studies. Vasc Health Risk Manag 2008;4:103–13.

19. Sato N, Kajimoto K, Asai K, et al. Acute decompensated heart failure syndromes (ATTEND) registry. A prospective observational multicenter cohort study: rationale, design, and preliminary data. Am Heart J 2010;159:949–55.e1.

20. Wang SS, Chu SH, Ko WJ. Clinical outcome of heart transplantation: experience at the National Taiwan University Hospital. Transplant Proc 1996;28:1733–4.

21. Chawalit O, Meunmai S, Kittichai L, et al. The first successful heart transplantation in South East Asia. Rinsho Kyobu Geka 1988;8:480–3.

22. Chu SH, Hsu RB, Wang SS. Heart transplantation in Asia. Ann Thorac Cardiovasc Surg 1999;5:361–4.

23. Ota K. Asian transplant registry. Transplant Proc 2004;36:1865–7.

24. Ota K. Asian transplant registry (1999). Transplant Proc 2001;33:1989–92.

25. Takagi H. Organ transplants still too few in Japan and Asian countries. Transplant Proc 1997;29:1580–3.

26. Cardiac transplantation in Hong Kong. The education corner. The Hong Kong Society of Transplantation. 2015. Available at: http://www.hkst.org/the-education-corner/57-cardiac-transplantation-in-hong-kong.html. Accessed April 30, 2015.

27. Chau E. Cardiac transplantation in Hong Kong. Hong Kong Medical Diary 2001;6:3.

28. Mahdavi-Mazdeh M, Rouchi AH, Rajolani H, et al. Transplantation registry in Iran. Transplant Proc 2008;40:126–8.

29. Mandegar MH, Bagheri J, Chitsaz S, et al. Heart transplantation in Iran: a comprehensive single-center review of 15-year performance. Arch Iran Med 2009;12:111–5.

30. Kitamura S. Heart transplantation in Japan: a critical appraisal for the results and future prospects. Gen Thorac Cardiovasc Surg 2012;60:639–44.

31. Nakatani T, Fukushima N, Ono M, et al. The registry report of heart transplantation in Japan (1999-2013). Circ J 2014;78:2604–9.

32. Cha MJ, Lee HY, Cho HJ, et al. Under-utilization of donor hearts in the initial era of the heart transplant program in Korea - review of 13 years' experience from the Korea national registry. Circ J 2013;77:2056–63.

33. Jung SH, Kim JJ, Choo SJ, et al. Long-term mortality in adult orthotopic heart transplant recipients. J Korean Med Sci 2011;26:599–603.

34. SCOT Data. Organ transplantation in Saudi Arabia–2013. Saudi J Kidney Dis Transpl 2014;25:1359–68.

35. Canver CC, Al Buraiki JA, Saad E, et al. A high-volume heart transplantation center in an Islamic country. Asian Cardiovasc Thorac Ann 2011;19:244–8.

36. Sivathasan C. Heart transplantation in Singapore. Ann Acad Med Singapore 2009;38:309–14.

37. Wang SS, Wang CH, Chou NK, et al. Current status of heart transplantation in Taiwan. Transplant Proc 2014;46:911–3.

38. Lee KF, Lin CY, Tsai YT, et al. The status of heart transplantation in Taiwan, 2005-2010. Transplant Proc 2014;46:934–6.

39. Ongcharit C, Ongcharit P. Intrathoracic organ transplantation in Thailand. Transplant Proc 1998;30:3385–6.

40. Heart surgery statistics by The Society of Thoracic Surgeons of Thailand. 2015. Available at: http://thaists.org/news_detail.php?news_id=212. Accessed May 30, 2015.

41. Nakatani T. Heart transplantation. Circ J 2009;73(Suppl A):A55–60.

42. Chen JW, Chen YS, Chi NH, et al. Risk factors and prognosis of patients with primary graft failure after heart transplantation: an Asian center experience. Transplant Proc 2014;46:914–9.

43. Chi NH, Chou NK, Yu YH, et al. Heart transplantation in end-stage rheumatic heart disease - experience of an endemic area. Circ J 2014;78:1900–7.

44. Yeom SY, Hwang HY, Oh SJ, et al. Heart transplantation in the elderly patients: midterm results. Korean J Thorac Cardiovasc Surg 2013;46:111–6.

45. Chen YC, Chuang MK, Chou NK, et al. Twenty-four year single-center experience of hepatitis B virus infection in heart transplantation. Transplant Proc 2012;44:910–2.

46. Chi NH, Chou NK, Tsao CI, et al. Endomyocardial biopsy in heart transplantation: schedule or event? Transplant Proc 2012;44:894–6.

47. Large S. Primary heart graft failure. Transplantation 2010;90:359.

48. Costanzo MR, Naftel DC, Pritzker MR, et al. Heart transplant coronary artery disease detected by coronary angiography: a multi-institutional study of pre-operative donor and recipient risk factors. Cardiac Transplant Research Database. J Heart Lung Transplant 1998;17:744–53.

49. Hsu RB, Chu SH, Wang SS, et al. Low incidence of transplant coronary artery disease in Chinese heart recipients. J Am Coll Cardiol 1999;33:1573–7.

50. Luo CM, Chou NK, Chi NH, et al. The effect of statins on cardiac allograft survival. Transplant Proc 2014;46:920–4.

51. Chang HY, Lo LW, Feng AN, et al. Long-term follow-up of arrhythmia characteristics and clinical

outcomes in heart transplant patients. Transplant Proc 2013;45:369–75.

52. Dasari TW, Pavlovic-Surjancev B, Patel N, et al. Incidence, risk factors, and clinical outcomes of atrial fibrillation and atrial flutter after heart transplantation. Am J Cardiol 2010;106:737–41.

53. Hsu RB, Chang CI, Tsai MK, et al. Low incidence of malignancy in heart-transplant recipients in Taiwan: an update and comparison with kidney-transplant recipients. Eur J Cardiothorac Surg 2010;37:1117–21.

54. Yin WY, Koo M, Lee MC, et al. Incidence of non-Hodgkin lymphomas and the ten most commonly diagnosed cancers after heart transplantation: a nationwide population-based study in Taiwan. Transplantation 2014;98:e71–3.

55. Chen CH, Shu KH, Ho HC, et al. A nationwide population-based study of the risk of tuberculosis in different solid organ transplantations in Taiwan. Transplant Proc 2014;46:1032–5.

56. Nishi H, Toda K, Miyagawa S, et al. Initial experience in Japan with HeartWare ventricular assist system. J Artif Organs 2014;17:149–56.

57. Deo SV, Sung K, Daly RC, et al. Cardiac transplantation after bridged therapy with continuous flow left ventricular assist devices. Heart Lung Circ 2014;23:224–8.

Epidemiology of Heart Failure in Asia

Naoki Sato, MD, PhD, FESC

KEYWORDS

- Hospitalized heart failure • Site selection • Time frame • Ethnicity
- Guideline-directed medical therapy • Mortality

KEY POINTS

- The following key issues regarding the comparison between epidemiologic studies should be considered: (1) definitions of heart failure (HF) in registries of patients hospitalized for HF, (2) site selection, (3) time frame, and (4) ethnic differences.
- Asian patients with HF are younger and more ethnically different, and the proportion of de novo cases is relatively higher in Asian patients with HF than in Western patients with HF.
- Asian patients with HF have still not received guideline-directed medical therapy (GDMT) well, especially β-blockers at discharge.
- The outcome of Asian patients with HF was poor and almost similar to that of Western patients with HF.

INTRODUCTION

HF is increasing in prevalence and is a public health problem in the Western countries as well as in Asia. The most critical issues of HF are high mortality and readmission rates. However, epidemiologic studies in Asia have not been well conducted to clarify the present status of HF management. From the overview of the studies regarding HF in Asia, the prevalence of HF is 1.2% to 6.7% depending on the population studied.[1–4] In China, there are 4.2 million patients with HF and 500,000 new cases are being diagnosed each year.[5] In Japan, it is estimated that there are 1.0 million patients with HF and the number of outpatients with left ventricular dysfunction is predicted to gradually increase to 1.3 million by 2030.[6] Thus, epidemiologic data for HF are essential to improve the incidence and outcome of HF. However, there are several concerns when the patient characteristics and management are compared among countries. Definitions of HF,

differences in sites, the time frame when the registry was performed, and ethnic differences should be clarified. Also, especially in Asia, the status of economic situation and life styles, which are quite different from those of Western countries and even between Asian countries, should be considered. Based on these considerations, the results of comparison of characteristics and management of patients with HF in Asian countries should be taken into account.

IMPORTANT ISSUES FOR EPIDEMIOLOGIC COMPARISON
Definitions of Heart Failure in Registries of Patients Hospitalized for Heart Failure

In HF registries, it is important to clarify the definition of HF. **Table 1** shows the definition of HF in representative registries of patients hospitalized for HF in the United States, Europe, and Asian countries.[7–13] Actually there are studies in which the definition of HF was not clarified.

Conflict of interest: none.
Cardiology and Intensive Care Unit, Nippon Medical School Musashi-Kosugi Hospital, 1-396 Kosugi-cho Naka-hara-ku, Kawasaki, Kanagawa 211-8533, Japan
E-mail address: nms-nd@nms.ac.jp

Heart Failure Clin 11 (2015) 573–579
http://dx.doi.org/10.1016/j.hfc.2015.07.009
1551-7136/15/$ – see front matter © 2015 Elsevier Inc. All rights reserved.

Table 1
Definition of HF in registries of patients hospitalized for HF

Study	Country or Region	Definition
ADHERE[7]	United States	ICD-9 codes related to HF
OPTIMIZE-HF[8]	United States	ICD-9 codes related to HF
EHFS II[9]	Europe	(1) Symptoms (dyspnea) and signs (ie, rales, hypotension, hypoperfusion, right ventricular HF) of HF and (2) lung congestion on chest radiograph
ADHERE International-Asia Pacific[10]	Asia Pacific (Singapore, Thailand, Indonesia, Australia, Malaysia, Philippines, Taiwan, Hong Kong)	ICD-9 or ICD-10 codes related to HF
KorHF registry[11]	Korea	Framingham criteria
KorAHF registry[12]	Korea	Signs or symptoms of HF and one of the following criteria are eligible for the study: (1) lung congestion or (2) objective findings of LV systolic dysfunction or structural heart disease. Lung congestion has been defined as congestion on a chest radiograph or as rales on physical examination
ATTEND registry[13]	Japan	Modified Framingham criteria

Abbreviations: ADHERE, Acute Decompensated Heart Failure National Registry; ATTEND, Acute Decompensated Heart Failure Syndromes; EHFS II, EuroHeart Failure Survey II; ICD, *International Classification of Diseases*; KorAHF, Korean Acute Heart Failure; LV, left ventricular; OPTIMIZE-HF, Organized Program to Initiate Lifesaving Treatment in Hospitalized Patients with Heart Failure.

Especially in the registries that include patients with HF with left ventricular preserved ejection fraction (HF-PEF), it is important to clarify the definition of HF-PEF. It will be meaningless to compare the data from the HF registries without the definition of HF. Furthermore, the interpretation of comparison between registries with different definitions of HF should be done with caution. Therefore, future registries should use the same definition of HF, such as the definition of HF suggested by the European Society of Cardiology Guidelines for the diagnosis and treatment of acute and chronic HF 2012.[14] The diagnosis of HF-reduced ejection fraction (EF) requires the following 3 conditions: (1) symptoms typical of HF, (2) signs typical of HF, and (3) reduced left ventricular (LVEF). The diagnosis of HF-PEF requires the following 4 conditions: (1) symptoms typical of HF, (2) signs typical of HF, (3) normal or only mildly reduced LVEF and left ventricle (LV) not dilated, and (4) relevant structural heart disease (LV hypertrophy/left auricular enlargement) and/or diastolic dysfunction. In the analysis of large database, for example, national database, the *International Classification of Diseases, Tenth Revision* (ICD-10) codes might be best to define HF.

Site Selection

Patient characteristics are different between sites. Site selection should be decided according to the aim of registry. In a registry collecting the real-world data of the patient characteristics and management in each country or region, balanced, which means that participating sites consist of both academic and nonacademic ones, sites and regions must be included. For example, in the Acute Decompensated Heart Failure National Registry (ADHERE), the sites were selected to represent academic and nonacademic ones as well as the well-balanced geographic regions of the United States.[7]

The Time Frame

The time frame when the registry was performed is also important for comparison of HF data between counties. In China, the causes of HF markedly changed during past 2 decades, that is, a decrease in the proportion of valvular heart disease due mainly to rheumatic fever and an increase in the proportion of ischemic heart disease.[15] Thus, the time frame should be considered for comparison between countries. On the other hand, the trends of characteristics and management of patients with HF is clinically valuable to improve the HF outcome in each country and region. From this viewpoint, periodic epidemiologic studies should be conducted.

Ethnic Differences

Ethnic differences are also another issue in international comparison of HF. In **Table 2**, the distribution of ethnic groups in each Asian country is shown.[16] In Singapore, the report of HF, defined by *ICD, Ninth Revision* (ICD-9) codes, from 1991 to 1998 revealed the ethnic differences, which showed higher hospital admission rates with both Malays and Indians than with Chinese and a rising mortality in Malays compared with other ethnic groups.[3] Thus in most Asian countries except China, South Korea, Thailand, and Japan, ethnic differences should be considered.

EPIDEMIOLOGIC COMPARISON OF PATIENTS HOSPITALIZED FOR HEART FAILURE IN ASIA
Patient Characteristics

The comparison of characteristics for representative patients hospitalized for HF is shown in **Table 3**.[4,5,9,17–20] The mean age of patients hospitalized for HF in Asian countries, except Japan, was less than those of Western countries, which can be explained by the differences in life expectancy, adult literacy, educational level, and standard of living.[10] Approximately 60% of patients hospitalized for HF in Asian countries were male, which was slightly higher than data from American registries, but was similar to those from the European registry. The proportions of ischemic cause were lower in Asian patients with HF than those in Western registries. This difference would be due in part to dietary habits. In China, ischemic and hypertensive causes of HF are becoming common, because of the decrease in rheumatic valvular diseases and the increasing wealth and improvement in socioeconomic conditions over the past 2 decades.[21] Interestingly, the proportions of patients with de novo HF in both Korea and Japan were higher than those in Western and other Asian countries. Patients with de novo HF commonly have hypertension and are admitted to the emergency room (ER) because of cardiogenic pulmonary edema with HF-PEF. However, the prevalence of HF with reduced EF in both Korea and Japan was consistent with prevalence in Western registries. Thus the reason for high prevalence of de novo HF is unknown, but it might be partly due to the differences in communication between ER physicians and cardiologists in the sites.

Management

During the acute phase after admission for HF, data regarding management are available only in Korean and Japanese registries,[12,19] but not in Chinese studies. A comparison of management during hospitalization is shown in **Table 4**.[9,12,17,19] Inotropes were more commonly used in both Europe and Korea than in the United States and Japan. The ADHERE registry did not include cardiogenic shock

Table 2	
Distribution of ethnic groups in Asian countries	
Country	**Ethnic Group Distribution (% of Total Population)**
China	Han Chinese (91.6%), Zhuang (1.3%), others (7.1%)
Indonesia	Javanese (40.1%), Sundanese (15.5%), Malay (3.7%), Batak (3.6%), Madurese (3%), Betawi (2.9%), Minangkabau (2.7%), Buginese (2.7%), Bantenese (2%), Banjarese (1.7%), Balinese (1.7%), Acehnese (1.4%), Dayak (1.4%), Sasak (1.3%), Chinese (1.2%), others (15%)
Japan	Japanese (98.5%), Koreans (0.5%), Chinese (0.4%), others (0.6%)
Korea, South	Homogeneous
Malaysia	Malay (50.1%), Chinese (22.6%), indigenous (11.8%), Indians (6.7%), others (0.7%), noncitizens (8.2%)
Philippines	Tagalog (28.1%), Cebuano (13.1%), Ilocano (9%), Bisaya/Binisaya (7.6%), Hiligaynon Ilonggo (7.5%), Bikol (6%), Waray (3.4%), others (25.3%)
Singapore	Chinese (74.2%), Malay (13.3%), Indians (9.2%), others (3.3%)
Thailand	Thai (95.9%), Burmese (2%), others (1.3%), unspecified (0.9%)
Vietnam	Kinh (Viet) (85.7%), Tay (1.9%), Thai (1.8%), Muong (1.5%), Khmer (1.5%), Mong (1.2%), Nung (1.1%), others (5.3%)

Data from Central Intelligence Agency. The world factbook. Available at: https://www.cia.gov/library/publications/the-world-factbook/fields/2075.html#71. Accessed July 7, 2015.

Table 3
Characteristics for representative patients hospitalized for HF

	ADHERE[17]	OPTIMIZE-HF[18]	EFHS II[19]	ATTEND[19]	KorAHF[12]	China[4,5,20]	ADHERE International[10]
Region	United States	United States	Europe	Japan	Korea, South	China report 2012, 42 hospitals	8 Asia Pacific countries
Time frame	2001–2004	2003–2004	2004–2005	2007–2012	2011	2000	2006–2008
N	105,388	48,612	3580	4842	2066 (May 2012)	6777	10,171
HF definition	ICD-9	ICD-9	Signs & symptoms + lung congestion	Framingham criteria	Signs & symptoms + lung congestion	—	ICD-9 or ICD-10
Age (y)	72 ± 14	73 ± 14	70 ± 13	73 ± 14	69 ± 14	68 ± 17	66
Males	48	48	61	58	55	—	57
Ischemic cause	—	46	54	31	38	45	—
Hypertensive cause	—	23	—	18	6	13	—
EF<40%	51	49	66 (<45%)	53	56	—	53
HTN	73	71	63	69	59	—	64
De novo HF	24	12	37	64	50	—	36
DM	44	42	33	34	36	—	45
Afib	31	31	39	40	27	—	24
COPD	31	15	19	10	11	—	—
HR (bpm)	—	87 ± 22	95	99 ± 29	91 ± 26 (pulse rate)	—	—
SBP (mm Hg)	144 ± 33	143 ± 33	135	146 ± 37	136 ± 31	—	—
Orthopnea	—	27	—	63	—	—	—
Edema	65	65	—	67	—	—	—
sCr levels (mg/dL)	1.8 ± 1.6	1.8 ± 1.8	—	1.4 ± 1.6	1.5 ± 1.6	—	—
BNP levels, (pg/mL)	840	832	—	707[a]	904[a]	—	—

Values are in %, mean ± standard deviation.
Abbreviations: Afib, atrial fibrillation; ATTEND, Acute Decompensated Heart Failure Syndromes; BNP, brain natriuretic peptide; COPD, chronic obstructive pulmonary disease; DM, diabetes mellitus; EF, ejection fraction; EHFS II, European heart failure survey II; HR, heart rate; HTN, hypertension; KorAHF, Korean Acute Heart Failure; OPTIMIZE-HF, Organized Program to Initiate Lifesaving Treatment in Hospitalized Patients with Heart Failure; SBP, systolic blood pressure; sCr, serum creatinine.
[a] Median.

Table 4
Intravenous therapies and nonpharmacologic treatments

	ADHERE[17]	EHFS II[9]	ATTEND[19]	KorAHF[12]
IV therapies				
Diuretics	92	84	76	72
Vasodilators	9	38	78	40
Inotropes	15	30	19	32
Nonpharmacologic therapies				
PCI	8	8	8	10
CABG	—	1.8	1.3	2.1
IABP	<1	2.2	2.5	3.9
Mechanical ventilation	5	5	7.5 (intubation)	3.6
Ultrafiltration	5	—	2.6[a]	4.3[a]

Values are in percentage
Abbreviations: CABG, coronary artery bypass graft; IABP, intra-aortic balloon pumping; IV, intravenous; PCI, percutaneous coronary intervention.
[a] Continuous renal replacement therapy.

of ICD-9 codes.[7] In the Acute Decompensated Heart Failure Syndromes (ATTEND) registry, the prevalence of hypotension defined as less than 100 mm Hg was 7.7%.[19] In the EuroHeart Failure Survey II (EHFS II) registry, cardiogenic shock was present in 3.9%.[9] The proportion of patients with low systolic blood pressure less than 90 mm Hg was 5% in the Korean Acute Heart Failure (KorAHF) registry.[12] Although there were no significant differences in systolic blood pressure among these registries, inotropes were commonly used in Europe and Korea. In the EHFS II registry, dobutamine, dopamine, levosimendan, and noradrenaline were used in 10.2%, 11.3%, 3.9%, and 2.6%, respectively.[9] In the KorAHF registry, dobutamine, dopamine, milrinone, and norepinephrine were used in 23.9%, 18.1%, 1.5%, and 7%, respectively.[12] Thus dobutamine was seen to be the most commonly used drug. Regarding nonpharmacologic treatments including supported circulatory devices, there were no significant differences between Western and Asian countries.

In **Fig. 1**, the prescriptions of oral medication at discharge are shown. The use of β-blockers in Asian countries, except Japan, was lower than that in Western countries. A Chinese retrospective survey of patients hospitalized for chronic systolic HF in 12 hospitals in Hubei province revealed that 52%, 19%, 47%, 46%, and 69% of patients (n = 16,681) were on angiotensin-converting enzyme inhibitors (ACEI), angiotensin II receptor blockers (ARB), β-blockers, digoxin, and diuretics, respectively, showing the low rate of prescription of β-blockers.[21] However, the recent study in China demonstrated the improvements of

pharmacologic therapies at discharge according to the GDMT, that is, ACEI/ARB, β-blockers, and aldosterone blockers were prescribed at the rates of 66%, 68%, and 74%, respectively.[22] The use of digoxin was around 30%, which was not different between Asia, except for Japan, and Western countries. Diuretics, mainly loop diuretics, were prescribed in 80% to 90% of both Asian and Western patients with HF. In these studies, there were no data regarding the doses of standard medication based on the GDMT. Future Asian epidemiologic studies should collect the information including the proportion receiving GDMT.

Outcome

The median length of stay was almost similar in most registries, that is, 4.3 days in ADHERE,[17] 9 days in EHFS II,[9] 8 days in KorAHF,[12] and 6 days in ADHERE International (Singapore, Thailand, Indonesia, Australia, Malaysia, Philippines, Taiwan, and Hong Kong).[10] However, a Chinese study in 42 hospitals (n = 6777) demonstrated that the hospital stay was 21.8 days in 2000.[20] In Japan, the median length of stay was 21 days.[19] Thus, the length of hospital stay was longer in both China and Japan than in other Asian countries. In Japan, these differences might be caused by the differences in the health insurance system, medical costs, and so on, but the exact reasons have not been clarified in China. From the viewpoint of safe length of stay, one suggestion was reported from the ATTEND. The frequency of sudden death was much higher during the first 14 days after admission than at any other time, with 71.4% of sudden deaths occurring during

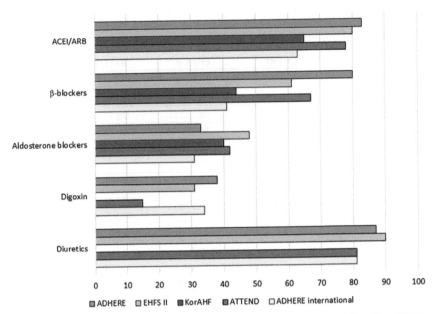

Fig. 1. Medication ad discharge in representative registries. In most Asian countries, the GDMT was not performed well, especially the use of β-blockers. Importantly, the present status regarding GDMT was clarified by the epidemiologic studies. Based on these results, the present status should be improved in each Asian country and then the improvement should be confirmed by the next epidemiologic study. Data for both digoxin and diuretics are not available in the KorAHF registry. ACEI, angiotensin converting enzyme inhibitors; ARB, angiotensin II receptor blockers.

this period.[23] Therefore, the appropriate length of stay might be 14 days.

In-hospital mortality was approximately 4% to 7% in Asian and Western registries, which was similar to that of acute myocardial infarction. However, middle or long-term outcomes of HF were poor in both Asian and Western countries. In the Atherosclerosis Risk in Communities (ARIC) study, the 30-day, 1-year, and 5-year case fatality rates after hospitalization for HF were 10.4%, 22%, and 42.3%, respectively.[24] Middle- and long-term mortalities in Western countries remain poor, although the survival rate has improved. In the KorAHF registry,[11] the cumulative survival rate after discharge at 1 year was 85%. The recent study in Korea, KorAHF registry, demonstrated that all-cause mortalities at 30 days and 180 days were 1.2% and 9.2% and HF readmission rates were 6.4% and 24%, respectively.[12] In Chinese patients with HF with reduced EF with dilated cardiomyopathy (DCM) and ischemic cardiomyopathy (ICM), the all-cause mortality and sudden cardiac death were higher in DCM than in ICM (47% vs 35% for all-cause mortality, and 17% vs 12% for sudden cardiac death).[22] In Japan, the length of stay was long, but the all-cause mortality was similar to that of the ARIC study.[24,25] Therefore, the critical issue regarding

outcome in patients hospitalized for HF exists in Asia as well as in Western countries.

SUMMARY

In Asia, epidemiologic data are still lacking in most countries. Registries for patients hospitalized for HF should be conducted as early as possible to improve the poor outcome in each Asian country. To clarify the differences between Asian countries or between Asian and Western countries, global epidemiologic studies based on the same protocol should be conducted.

REFERENCES

1. Chong AY, Rajaratnam R, Hussein NR, et al. Heart failure in a multiethnic population in Kuala Lumpur, Malaysia. Eur J Heart Fail 2003;5:569–74.
2. Guo Y, Lip GY, Banerjee A. Heart failure in East Asia. Curr Cardiol Rev 2013;9:112–22.
3. Ng TP, Niti M, Tan WC. Trends and ethnic differences in asthma hospitalization rates in Singapore, 1991 to 1998. Ann Allergy Asthma Immunol 2003;90:51–5.
4. Yang YN, Ma YT, Liu F, et al. Incidence and distributing feature of chronic heart failure in adult population of Xinjiang. Zhonghua Xin Xue Guan Bing Za Zhi 2010;38:460–4 [in Chinese].

5. Hu SS, Kong LZ, Gao RL, et al. Outline of the report on cardiovascular disease in China, 2010. Biomed Environ Sci 2012;25:251–6.

6. Okura Y, Ramadan MM, Ohno Y, et al. Impending epidemic: future projection of heart failure in Japan to the year 2055. Circ J 2008;72:489–91.

7. Adams KF Jr, Fonarow GC, Emerman CL, et al, ADHERE Scientific Advisory Committee and Investigators. Characteristics and outcomes of patients hospitalized for heart failure in the United States: rationale, design, and preliminary observations from the first 100,000 cases in the Acute Decompensated Heart Failure National Registry (ADHERE). Am Heart J 2005;149:209–16.

8. Fonarow GC, Abraham WT, Albert NM, et al. Organized Program to Initiate Lifesaving Treatment in Hospitalized Patients with Heart Failure (OPTI-MIZE-HF): rationale and design. Am Heart J 2004; 148:43–51.

9. Nieminen MS, Brutsaert D, Dickstein K, et al, Euro-Heart Survey Investigators. EuroHeart Failure Survey II (EHFS II): a survey on hospitalized acute heart failure patients: description of population. Eur Heart J 2006;27:2725–36.

10. Atherton JJ, Hayward CS, Wan Ahmad WA, et al, ADHERE International–Asia Pacific Scientific Advisory Committee. Patient characteristics from a regional multicenter database of Acute Decompensated Heart Failure in Asia Pacific (ADHERE International-Asia Pacific). J Card Fail 2012;18:82–8.

11. Choi DJ, Han S, Jeon ES, et al, KorHF Registry. Characteristics, outcomes and predictors of long-term mortality for patients hospitalized for acute heart failure: a report from the Korean Heart Failure registry. Korean Circ J 2011;41:363–71.

12. Lee SE, Cho HJ, Lee HY, et al. A multicentre cohort study of acute heart failure syndromes in Korea: rationale, design, and interim observations of the Korean Acute Heart Failure (KorAHF) registry. Eur J Heart Fail 2014;16:700–8.

13. Sato N, Kajimoto K, Asai K, et al, ATTEND Investigators. Acute Decompensated Heart Failure Syndromes (ATTEND) registry. A prospective observational multicenter cohort study: rationale, design, and preliminary data. Am Heart J 2010;159:949–55.

14. McMurray JJ, Adamopoulos S, Anker SD, et al, ESC Committee for Practice Guidelines. ESC Guidelines for the diagnosis and treatment of acute and chronic heart failure 2012: the Task force for the diagnosis and treatment of acute and chronic heart failure 2012 of the European Society of Cardiology. Developed in collaboration with the Heart Failure Association (HFA) of the ESC. Eur Heart J 2012;33: 1787–847.

15. Ariely R, Evans K, Mills T. Heart failure in China: a review of the literature. Drugs 2013;73:689–701.

16. Central Intelligence Agency. The world factbook. Available at: https://www.cia.gov/library/publications/the-world-factbook/fields/2075.html#71. Accessed July 27, 2015.

17. Fonarow GC, Heywood JT, Heidenreich PA, et al, ADHERE Scientific Advisory Committee and Investigators. Temporal trends in clinical characteristics, treatments, and outcomes for heart failure hospitalizations, 2002 to 2004: findings from Acute Decompensated Heart Failure National Registry (ADHERE). Am Heart J 2007;153:1021–8.

18. Abraham WT, Fonarow GC, Albert NM, et al, OPTI-MIZE-HF Investigators and Coordinators. Predictors of in-hospital mortality in patients hospitalized for heart failure: insights from the Organized Program to Initiate Lifesaving Treatment in Hospitalized Patients with Heart Failure (OPTIMIZE-HF). J Am Coll Cardiol 2008;52:347–56.

19. Sato N, Kajimoto K, Keida T, et al, ATTEND Investigators. Clinical features and outcome in hospitalized heart failure in Japan (from the ATTEND registry). Circ J 2013;77:944–51.

20. Zhang J. Report on cardiovascular diseases in China 2012. Heart failure. Chin Med J 2014; 127(Suppl 2):79–82.

21. Society of Cardiology, Chinese Medical Association. Retrospective investigation of hospitalized patients with heart failure in some parts of China in 1980, 1990, 2000. Chin J Cardiol 2002;30:450–4. Available at: http://eng.med.wanfangdata.com.cn/JournalSingle.aspx?qkID=zhxxgb&year=2002&issue=08. Accessed July 27, 2015.

22. Liu X, Yu H, Pei J, et al. Clinical characteristics and long-term prognosis in patients with chronic heart failure and reduced ejection fraction in China. Heart Lung Circ 2014;23:818–26.

23. Kajimoto K, Sato N, Keida T, et al, Investigators of the Acute Decompensated Heart Failure Syndromes (ATTEND) Registry. Association between length of stay, frequency of in-hospital death, and causes of death in Japanese patients with acute heart failure syndromes. Int J Cardiol 2013;168:554–6.

24. Loehr LR, Rosamond WD, Chang PP, et al. Heart failure incidence and survival (from the Atherosclerosis Risk in Communities study). Am J Cardiol 2008;101: 1016–22.

25. Kajimoto K, Sato N, Takano T, Investigators of the Acute Decompensated Heart Failure Syndromes (ATTEND) Registry. Association of age and baseline systolic blood pressure with outcomes in patients hospitalized for acute heart failure syndromes. Int J Cardiol 2015;191:100–6.

Identifying Barriers and Practical Solutions to Conducting Site-Based Research in North America
Exploring Acute Heart Failure Trials As a Case Study

Andrew P. Ambrosy, MD[a],*, Robert J. Mentz, MD[a,b],
Arun Krishnamoorthy, MD[a,b], Stephen J. Greene, MD[a],
Harry W. Severance, MD[c]

KEYWORDS

- Acute heart failure • Clinical trials • Site-based research

KEY POINTS

- There are more than 1 million hospitalizations for acute heart failure annually in the United States accounting for most of the $40 billion spent directly on HF-related care.
- Although the treatment and prognosis of ambulatory HF patients has improved dramatically because of drug- and device-based therapies, there have been few advancements in the management of AHF and postdischarge readmissions and mortality remain unacceptably high.
- One of the emerging trends in global clinical trials has been the gradual shift of enrollment from predominantly North America and Western Europe to Eastern Europe, South America, and Asia-Pacific where the regulatory burden and cost of conducting research may be less prohibitive.
- The crisis in site-based research in North America is exacerbated by poor visibility of cardiovascular disease and clinical trials, an inability to identify highly performing centers in terms of volume and quality, time-consuming study protocols not reflective of the realities of patient care, inadequate infrastructure for recruitment and study conduct, underdeveloped relationships between the research team and emergency providers and hospital-based physicians, misaligned incentives between principle investigators and the parent clinical facilities, and limited training and support for study coordinators.

Disclosures: Dr R.J. Mentz receives research support from the NIH, Amgen, AstraZeneca, Bristol-Myers Squibb, GlaxoSmithKline, Gilead, Novartis, Otsuka, and ResMed; honoraria from Novartis, Thoratec, and HeartWare; and has served on an advisory board for Luitpold Pharmaceuticals, Inc. Dr A. Krishnamoorthy reports working on projects funded by research grants to the Duke Clinical Research Institute from the NIH, Novartis, Daiichi-Sankyo, Eli Lilly, and Maquet and support to attend educational conferences from HeartWare and Medtronic. All other authors have no conflicts of interest to declare.

[a] Division of Cardiology, Duke University School of Medicine, 2301 Erwin Road Drive, Durham, NC 27710, USA;
[b] Division of Cardiology, Duke Clinical Research Institute, 2301 Erwin Road Drive, Durham, NC 27710, USA;
[c] Erlanger Institute for Clinical Research, 973 E. 3rd St. Ste B1203, Chattanooga, TN 37403, USA
* Corresponding author. Division of Cardiology, Duke University Medical Center, 2301 Erwin Road Drive, Durham, NC 27710.
E-mail address: andrew.ambrosy@dm.duke.edu

Heart Failure Clin 11 (2015) 581–589
http://dx.doi.org/10.1016/j.hfc.2015.07.002
1551-7136/15/$ – see front matter © 2015 Elsevier Inc. All rights reserved.

INTRODUCTION

There are approximately 6 million patients with heart failure (HF) in the United States with the prevalence projected to exceed 8 million by the year 2030.[1,2] In addition, there are more than 1 million hospital admissions annually in the United States accounting for most of the approximately $40 billion in direct costs for HF-related care each year. Following an index hospitalization for HF, the risk of readmission and death, respectively, may be 30% and 15% within 60 to 90 days.[3] Although the treatment of ambulatory HF has been revolutionized by drug- and device-based therapies over the past few decades, inpatient management has remained virtually unchanged over a similar time frame and nearly every clinical trial conducted to date has been neutral in terms of efficacy and/or safety.

The reasons for the lack of success with prior clinical trial programs is likely multifactorial and may be caused by issues related to the study drug and the target patient population (**Fig. 1**).[4] However, more recently, problems with study execution and enrollment at the level of the trial site and geographic region have received increasing attention. One of the emerging trends in global clinical trials has been the gradual shift of enrollment from predominantly North America and Western Europe to Eastern Europe, South America, and Asia-Pacific where the regulatory burden and cost of conducting research may be less prohibitive (**Table 1**). However, major regional differences in patient characteristics, background therapy, and event rates (ie, rehospitalizations and mortality)

may limit the generalizability of research conducted exclusively outside of North America to the US patient population.[5–7] This article uses acute HF (AHF) as a paradigm and identifies barriers and practical solutions to successfully conducting site-based research (SBR) in North America (**Table 2**).

BARRIER: POOR VISIBILITY OF CARDIOVASCULAR DISEASE AND CLINICAL TRIALS WITHIN THE INSTITUTION AND THE BROADER COMMUNITY

Cardiovascular disease (CVD) is the number one cause of morbidity and mortality worldwide killing more patients than all cancers combined.[1] In addition, in the developing world the burden of CVD continues to grow because of increased life expectancy as a result of improved sanitation, socioeconomic advancement, and the decline in deaths caused by communicable diseases. Similarly, because of aging of the population and the success of medical therapy, the number of patients worldwide with HF is growing at a truly exponential rate with estimates of the global prevalence approaching 40 million.[8] However, compared with the pandemic proportions of HF-related morbidity and mortality, there is disproportionately low visibility among medical professionals and the general public. In contrast to many common cancers, there are few major not-for-profit organizations, outside of medical professional groups, or philanthropic fundraising efforts targeting CVD in general and HF in specific. Moreover, as compared with HF, patients

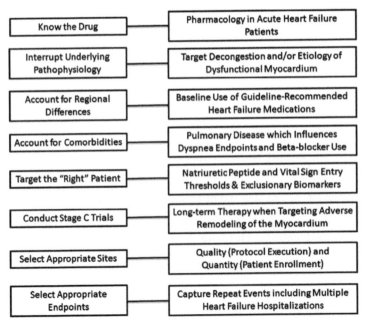

Fig. 1. Considerations for the successful design and conduct of acute heart failure trials. (*Adapted from* Mentz RJ. Learning from recent trials and shaping the future of acute heart failure trials. Am Heart J 2013;166(4):632; with permission.)

Know the Drug	Pharmacology in Acute Heart Failure Patients
Interrupt Underlying Pathophysiology	Target Decongestion and/or Etiology of Dysfunctional Myocardium
Account for Regional Differences	Baseline Use of Guideline-Recommended Heart Failure Medications
Account for Comorbidities	Pulmonary Disease which Influences Dyspnea Endpoints and Beta-blocker Use
Target the "Right" Patient	Natriuretic Peptide and Vital Sign Entry Thresholds & Exclusionary Biomarkers
Conduct Stage C Trials	Long-term Therapy when Targeting Adverse Remodeling of the Myocardium
Select Appropriate Sites	Quality (Protocol Execution) and Quantity (Patient Enrollment)
Select Appropriate Endpoints	Capture Repeat Events including Multiple Heart Failure Hospitalizations

Table 1
North American enrollment in recent acute heart failure trials

Trial	Year Published	Patient Population	Total Enrollment	North American Enrollment	% Enrolled in North American Sites
EVEREST	2007	Hospitalized HFrEF	4133	1251	30
ASCEND-HF	2011	Hospitalized HFrEF and HFpEF	7007	3149	45
RELAX-AHF	2013	Hospitalized HFrEF and HFpEF	1161	114	10
ASTRONAUT	2013	Hospitalized HFrEF	1615	124	8
Total	—	—	13,916	4638	33

Abbreviations: ASCEND-HF, Acute Study of Clinical Effectiveness of Nesiritide in Decompensated Heart Failure Trial; ASTRONAUT, The Aliskiren Trial on Acute Heart Failure Outcomes; EVEREST, Efficacy of Vasopressin Antagonism in Heart Failure: Outcomes Study with Tolvaptan; HFpEF, heart failure preserved ejection fraction; HFrEF, heart failure reduced ejection fraction; RELAX-AHF, A Study of Serelaxin Versus Placebo in Acute Heart Failure.
Adapted from Harinstein ME. Site selection for heart failure clinical trials in the USA. Heart Fail Rev 2015;20(4):377; with permission.

with cancer are generally more aware of their therapeutic options and prognosis, and oncologists reiterate that clinical trials may offer the one possible solution.[9] Thus, a logical first step in improving AHF trial participation in North America may be increasing provider and public awareness of the scope of the problem and the attendant morbidity and mortality.

BARRIER: INABILITY OF STUDY SPONSORS TO IDENTIFY SITES CAPABLE OF ENROLLING HIGH VOLUME AND QUALITY PATIENTS

Perhaps the single greatest impediment to expanding clinical trial enrollment in the United States is identifying sites capable of recruiting high volumes of patients without sacrificing quality in terms of violating inclusion/exclusion criteria, premature protocol termination, and lost to follow-up. For example, in the EVEREST (Efficacy of Vasopressin Antagonism in Heart Failure: Outcome Study with Tolvaptan) trial, there was a median per-site enrollment of six patients (range, 0–75) at 436 participating centers.[10] Seventy-seven sites did not enroll a single patient and more than 60% of sites enrolled less than or equal to 10 patients. Furthermore, the highest proportion of sites failing to enroll any patients was in North America and although North American sites represented 48% of total sites, they only contributed to 30% of overall enrollment (**Fig. 2**). Finally, higher and lower enrolling sites differed significantly in terms of baseline characteristics, protocol completion, and outcomes.

Table 2
Barriers and practical solutions to conducting site-based research in North America

Barrier	Practical Solutions
Poor visibility of cardiovascular disease and clinical trials within the institution and the broader community	Improve awareness
Inability of study sponsors to identify sites capable of enrolling high volume and quality patients	Pretrial registry
Time-consuming study protocols that do not reflect the day-to-day realities of patient care	Pragmatic trials
Inadequate infrastructure for recruitment of participants and study conduct	Clinical trial networks
Underdeveloped relationships between cardiologists and other physicians caring for the cardiac patient	Multispecialty collaborations
Misalignment of incentives between principle investigators and parent clinical facility	The research RVU
Limited upfront training and ongoing support for study coordinators and other staff	Site-based support

Abbreviation: RVU, relative value unit.

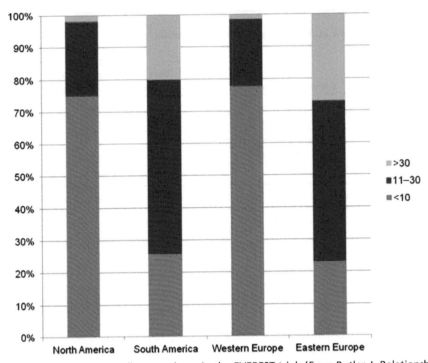

Fig. 2. Regional variation in site enrollment volume in the EVEREST trial. (*From* Butler J. Relationship between clinical trial site enrollment with participant characteristics, protocol completion, and outcomes: insights from the EVEREST (Efficacy of Vasopressin Antagonism in Heart Failure: Outcome Study with Tolvaptan) trial. J Am Coll Cardiol 2013;61(5):573.)

Although SBR is currently in a state of crisis in the United States, it is important to keep in mind that in the EVEREST trial, there were centers with relatively higher enrollment scattered throughout the world. Identifying these high-enrolling sites, while maintaining sufficient quality control, remains the goal of future drug development programs. It has been proposed that a pretrial registry may serve as a screening tool for subsequent trial participation (**Boxes 1** and **2**).[11–13] Incorporating a pretrial registry would allow investigators the opportunity to preview patient characteristics, evaluate protocol adherence, and estimate study enrollment. This up-front investment may facilitate study execution and be modest in comparison with the costs of maintaining poorly performing sites and conducting unsuccessful clinical trials. A global registry is currently underway that may integrate the pretrial paradigm on a global scale and inform future clinical development programs.[14]

BARRIER: TIME-CONSUMING STUDY PROTOCOLS THAT DO NOT REFLECT THE DAY-TO-DAY REALITIES OF PATIENT CARE

One of the major concerns raised by site-based researchers is that patient recruitments in AHF trials often disrupt the usual flow of patient care.

First, AHF trials have a high ratio of screened to enrolled patients because signs and symptoms of HF are neither sensitive nor specific and it is often too difficult to distinguish true "AHF" from "undifferentiated dyspnea" in the urgent or emergent setting.[15] In contrast, other CVD states, such as acute coronary syndrome (ACS), have a common pathophysiologic substrate (ie, plaque rupture and thrombosis) and clear presentation (ie, crushing substernal chest pain, electrocardiogram changes, and biomarker release) facilitating diagnosis and enrollment at the point-of-care. As a result, ACS trials have been able to rapidly and efficiently recruit thousands to tens of thousands of patients over a relatively shorter timeframe.

Second, AHF trials often use restrictive inclusion/exclusion criteria to enrich the study population for a homogenous group of patients more likely to respond favorably to study drug administration.[16] For example, one recent study applied the entry criteria for the RELAX-AHF (The Relaxin for the Treatment of Acute Heart Failure) trial to the ADHERE-U.S. (Acute Decompensated Heart Failure National Registry) and ADHERE-International registries and found that only approximately 2 in 10 patients with AHF in the United States, Latin America, or Asia-Pacific would have been eligible for enrollment.[17] Finally, AHF trials often include a

Box 1
Advantages of pretrial registries for appropriate site selection

Understand the disease characteristics in the intended study population

- Demographic variables (ie, age, gender, ethnicity)
- Distribution of heart failure causes and precipitating factors
  - Coronary artery disease versus other causes
  - Precipitating causes (ie, acute coronary syndromes, hypertension, atrial fibrillation, infectious causes, noncompliance)
- Heart failure treatment
  - Adherence to guidelines for medical treatment
  - Adherence to for device implantations
- Clinical course of the disease
  - Presentation (ie, signs, symptoms, clinical parameters)
  - Speed of symptom control and acute therapy that was administered to achieve this effect
  - Length of the hospital stay (including intensive care unit stay)
  - Procedures (ie, right or left heart catheterization, echocardiogram, balloon pump)
  - Discharge to rehabilitation/palliative care/other structures
- Event rate and general outcomes
  - Mortality, readmission, health care resource utilization rates
  - Causes of death and readmission: cardiovascular versus noncardiovascular

Estimate the power requirements of the study with respect to outcomes

- Estimate event rate to ensure study is adequately powered
- Ensure that the planned effect-size is clinically relevant
- Estimate variability in biomarker levels and other potential surrogate end points (ie, variation in laboratory cut-offs, comparability of assays, or genetics of patient population)
- Assess potential impact of protocol implementation on outcomes (ie, following a protocol might improve outcomes compared with institutional practice even in the placebo arm)

Improve protocol execution

- Center training: Allow time for better understanding of the process and terminology, including data recording and sample collection, detecting issues with language barriers and translation, and improving communication with coordinators
- Identify underperforming centers: Detect inadequate follow-up or compliance issues; corrective efforts can be used or center might be excluded from participation
- Predict enrollment rate in trial: Help guide whether enrollment rate will be adequate to achieve desired power within planned timeline
- Decreases chances of missing effective therapy

From Greene SJ. Designing effective drug and device development programs for hospitalized heart failure: a proposal for pretrial registries. Am Heart J 2014;168(2):146; with permission.

more prolonged duration of follow-up requiring a greater number of postdischarge visits and/or telephone contact. As a result, for all of the aforementioned reasons, patient recruitment and protocol adherence for many AHF trials may be an onerous undertaking at the site level for principle investigators and study coordinators.

In response to these concerns, several prominent clinical investigators have called for pragmatic trials to streamline recruitment and facilitate data collection. The prototypical example of this concept is the ASCEND-HF (Acute Study of Clinical Effectiveness of Nesiritide in Decompensated Heart Failure) trial, which was conducted to evaluate the efficacy

---

Box 2
Optimal center characteristics for successful participation in a multicenter trial

Proper patient enrollment

- Center achieves and maintains a high enrollment rate
- Patient characteristics conform to the enrollment criteria of the trial

High quality in protocol implementation and data collection

- Adherence to protocol process with minimal violations
- Adequate quality of collected data (minimal rates of missing data, verifiable from original sources with high fidelity of transcription, and so forth)

Good clinical practice in heart failure management

- Management of heart failure adheres to the current guideline-driven standards
  - Optimal medical treatment
  - Evidence-based device implantation (with consideration of regional variations in guidelines)
- Adequate documentation of diagnostic and therapeutic procedures

Patient follow-up procedures

- Established follow-up process
- Little or no loss to follow-up
- High-quality data on outcomes and adverse events (adjudication of outcomes)

From Greene SJ. Designing effective drug and device development programs for hospitalized heart failure: a proposal for pretrial registries. Am Heart J 2014;168(2):146; with permission.

---

and safety of nesiritide in AHF.[18,19] Enrollment criteria were broadly applicable including patients greater than or equal to 18 years of age hospitalized for an objective episode of AHF and primarily excluding patients with other life-limiting comorbidities or high-risk features and/or concomitant therapies precluding the provision of nesiritide. Study participants were randomized to a continuous infusion of nesiritide or placebo with or without an initial bolus for a minimum of 24 hours and a maximum of 7 days. Coprimary end points were dyspnea at 6 or 24 hours after study drug initiation and the composite of HF rehospitalization and death at 30 days. Thus, although nesiritide was ultimately found to be safe but no more efficacious than placebo, the ASCEND-HF trial, the largest conducted in AHF to date, is particularly noteworthy for taking a practical approach to trial design and conduct. These features may have contributed to the robust North American representation, with almost 50% of enrollment occurring in the United States and Canada.

BARRIER: INADEQUATE INFRASTRUCTURE FOR RECRUITMENT OF PARTICIPANTS AND STUDY CONDUCT

Few SBR organizations have a full-time research team. More commonly, principle investigators participate *ad hoc* in clinical trials based on interest and availability. In addition, study coordinators may include part-time or shared staffing models and clinical research activities are carried out simultaneously in the same physical space as standard of care. Study protocols may also have to go through the same cumbersome local institutional review board approval procedure at every single site. This slow and inefficient startup process occurs at a substantial premium and must be absorbed by the study sponsor and/or participating center. In addition, whether enrollment goals are met or not there are ongoing costs associated with keeping sites active.

A potential work-around is to establish permanent clinical trial networks with shared administrative overhead and dedicated research staff. In the purest form, industry and other sponsors would be able to approach a fully integrated academic or contract research organization with the authority to negotiate and make decisions on behalf of the entire network to simultaneously open enrollment across many individual and geographically diverse sites. In-network centers would be expected to have expedited start-up time and support staff with superior research training and specialized competency within various CVD states. There are many examples of existing multicenter research collaborations including the National Institutes of Health Heart Failure Network and the Duke University Cooperative Cardiovascular Society yet there are no large-scale, fully integrated clinical trial networks with the capacity to independently conduct pivotal studies across the spectrum of CVD on demand for potential sponsors.

BARRIER: UNDERDEVELOPED RELATIONSHIPS BETWEEN CARDIOLOGISTS AND OTHER PHYSICIANS CARING FOR THE CARDIAC PATIENT

There are more than 1 million admissions annually in the United States accounting for nearly 6.5 million hospital days.[1] It has been estimated that approximately 80% of patients with AHF initially present to the emergency room.[20] As a result, emergency physicians make all of the early decisions regarding diagnostic work-up and treatment. Emergency providers are also ultimately responsible for deciding disposition (ie, discharge vs admit) and triage (ie, observation, floor, telemetry, intensive care unit). In addition, with the growth of hospital-based medicine many patients admitted for AHF are being treated exclusively by internal medicine–trained hospitalists or in consultation with specialists in general cardiology and/or HF. However, despite the prominent role played by emergency physicians and hospitalists in the care of patients with AHF, these providers have traditionally been excluded from leadership roles at the site level, and clinical trials have historically relied on cardiology-based research teams to enroll patients up to 24 to 48 hours after hospital admission.

Thus, by excluding emergency physicians and hospitalists from participation in AHF trials, a significant number of potential participants may be outright missed and the enrollment of many more patients may be substantially delayed.[21,22] However, trial experience in such diverse diseases and conditions as ACS, sepsis, stroke, and trauma suggest that it is practical to enroll patients in the emergency room. In addition to direct referrals from emergency room staff, the research team may review admission logs, screen the electronic medical record remotely, or activate via automated alerts (ie, chief complaint, diagnosis, symptoms, laboratory values, and so forth). Although establishing a definitive diagnosis of AHF may theoretically be challenging in an urgent/emergent setting, several small-scale multicenter registries and trials have shown that it is feasible to diagnose and treat AHF within 6 to 12 hours of initial presentation.[15,23] Hence, it is imperative to build a collaborative relationship with emergency room physicians and hospital-based physicians at the site level to shift enrollment to the emergency department and the acute phase of hospitalization. This early enrollment may be critical to trial success depending on the study drug mechanism of action and the study end point. For example, in the URGENT-dyspnea study, greater than 75% of patients with AHF reported dyspnea improvement with standard therapy within 6 hours of emergency room presentation. Thus, for trials including dyspnea improvement as a primary end point, early recruitment in the emergency department may be critical to trial success.

BARRIER: MISALIGNMENT OF INCENTIVES BETWEEN PRINCIPLE INVESTIGATORS AND PARENT CLINICAL FACILITY

It is hard to make generalizations regarding the incentives for performing SBR because there is so much potential diversity in the relationship between the principle investigator and the parent clinical facility. For instance, the principle investigator's relationship with the parent clinical facility may range from being the sole proprietor or part of an ownership group to being a salaried employee. However, as a result of health care reform legislation and market trends, most clinical providers are now employees of academic or community-based hospitals and health care systems and they are often compensated for clinical services using formulas based on relative value units. Although the operating facility is often reimbursed at a premium for participating in clinical trials (ie, sponsor payments exceed normal payer mix, which would otherwise include lower payments from Medicaid and Medicare programs), clinician-investigators are often not compensated for time spent on research. Thus, clinician-investigators may paradoxically be compensated less for participating in SBR, whereas clinical trials may increase facility revenues directly by favorably changing the payer mix and indirectly by increasing the volume of patients seen and services rendered (ie, diagnostic testing, procedures, and so forth associated with study participation). A practical solution to realign incentives between site-based investigators and the parent clinical facility is to develop a research relative value unit to properly compensate providers for time and effort spent on clinical research. Furthermore, achievements in SBR may also be recognized by the institution for overall career advancement including promotions and consideration for tenure.

BARRIER: LIMITED UPFRONT TRAINING AND ONGOING SUPPORT FOR STUDY COORDINATORS AND OTHER STAFF

Although clinical trials are often led by a steering committee of academic and industry experts with substantial experience in the design and conduct of global research studies, most enrollment takes place at community-based, nonacademic hospitals and clinics. The local principle investigator and study coordinator usually are only able to devote part of their effort to SBR and may have variable prior experience and training. The research team is often provided with educational materials including background information, such as guideline-based recommendations for management and the rationale for the study. In addition, in some instances there may be in-person investigator meetings and/or telephone or World Wide Web conferences.

Industry sponsors often do not have the available personnel and infrastructure to manage the day-to-day aspects of a conducting a pivotal trial and must therefore rely on the assistance of academic research organizations or contract research organizations for site support, data collection, event adjudication, and data and safety monitoring. However, following a trial launch there may be very little contact between the study sponsor/academic leadership and site-based researchers. Furthermore, study coordinator may have little external or internal support to excel at SBR. It is obligatory for study sponsors, academic leaders, and academic research organizations/contract research organizations to monitor enrollment and prioritize the early troubleshooting of potential problems a priority. The sponsor may also further engage the local principle investigator and study coordinator by recognizing recruitment meeting or exceeding benchmarks with leadership roles in the trial and/or involvement in subsequent scientific publications.[24]

SUMMARY

AHF is a growing public health problem of pandemic proportions and there is currently an unmet need to expand the available therapeutic armamentarium. However, nearly every clinical trial conducted in AHF to date has been neutral in terms of efficacy and/or safety. In addition, SBR in North America is currently in a state of crisis with many trials being conducted predominantly or entirely in Eastern Europe, South America, and Asia-Pacific where patient characteristics, background therapy, and event rates may differ tremendously therefore limiting the generalizability to US patient populations. Although there is not a single panacea for remedying the decline in SBR in the United States, a combination of improving awareness of AHF and clinical trial opportunities, using registry data to preview patient characteristics and protocol adherence, designing and conducting pragmatic trials, establishing permanent clinical trial networks, building multispecialty collaborations to care for the cardiac patient, aligning financial incentives between clinician-investigators and hospital administrators by compensating for time and effort spent on research, and expanding start-up and ongoing site-based support may facilitate enrollment. Despite these global recommendations, improving the provider and patient experience in SBR in North America will ultimately require a more nuanced approach that implements changes at the site level and accounts for the uniqueness of each individual participating center.

REFERENCES

1. Mozaffarian D, Benjamin EJ, Go AS, et al. Heart disease and stroke statistics–2015 update: a report from the American Heart Association. Circulation 2015;131(4):e29–322.
2. Heidenreich PA, Albert NM, Allen LA, et al. Forecasting the impact of heart failure in the United States: a policy statement from the American Heart Association. Circ Heart Fail 2013;6(3):606–19.
3. Gheorghiade M, Abraham WT, Albert NM, et al. Systolic blood pressure at admission, clinical characteristics, and outcomes in patients hospitalized with acute heart failure. JAMA 2006;296(18):2217–26.
4. Butler J, Fonarow GC, Gheorghiade M. Strategies and opportunities for drug development in heart failure. JAMA 2013;309(15):1593–4.
5. Ambrosy AP, Fonarow GC, Butler J, et al. The global health and economic burden of hospitalizations for heart failure: lessons learned from hospitalized heart failure registries. J Am Coll Cardiol 2014;63(12):1123–33.
6. Ambrosy AP, Gheorghiade M, Chioncel O, et al. Global perspectives in hospitalized heart failure: regional and ethnic variation in patient characteristics, management, and outcomes. Curr Heart Fail Rep 2014;11(4):416–27.
7. Mentz RJ, Kaski JC, Dan GA, et al. Implications of geographical variation on clinical outcomes of cardiovascular trials. Am Heart J 2012;164(3):303–12.
8. Braunwald E. The war against heart failure: the *Lancet* lecture. Lancet 2015;385(9970):812–24.
9. Butler J, Fonarow GC, Gheorghiade M. Need for increased awareness and evidence-based therapies for patients hospitalized for heart failure. JAMA 2013;310(19):2035–6.

10. Butler J, Subacius H, Vaduganathan M, et al. Relationship between clinical trial site enrollment with participant characteristics, protocol completion, and outcomes: insights from the EVEREST (Efficacy of Vasopressin Antagonism in Heart Failure: Outcome Study with Tolvaptan) trial. J Am Coll Cardiol 2013;61(5):571–9.

11. Harinstein ME, Butler J, Greene SJ, et al. Site selection for heart failure clinical trials in the USA. Heart Fail Rev 2015;20(4):375–83.

12. Gheorghiade M, Vaduganathan M, Greene SJ, et al. Site selection in global clinical trials in patients hospitalized for heart failure: perceived problems and potential solutions. Heart Fail Rev 2014;19(2):135–52.

13. Greene SJ, Shah AN, Butler J, et al. Designing effective drug and device development programs for hospitalized heart failure: a proposal for pretrial registries. Am Heart J 2014;168(2):142–9.

14. Filippatos G, Khan SS, Ambrosy AP, et al. International REgistry to assess medical Practice with lOngitudinal obseRvation for Treatment of Heart Failure (REPORT-HF): rationale for and design of a global registry. Eur J Heart Fail 2015;17(5):527–33.

15. Mebazaa A, Pang PS, Tavares M, et al. The impact of early standard therapy on dyspnoea in patients with acute heart failure: the URGENT-dyspnoea study. Eur Heart J 2010;31(7):832–41.

16. Krishnamoorthy A, Tonks RW, Adams PA, et al. Enrollment in heart failure clinical trials: insights into which entry criteria exclude patients. J Card Fail 2015. [Epub ahead of print].

17. Wang TS, Hellkamp AS, Patel CB, et al. Representativeness of RELAX-AHF clinical trial population in acute heart failure. Circ Cardiovasc Qual Outcomes 2014;7(2):259–68.

18. Hernandez AF, O'Connor CM, Starling RC, et al. Rationale and design of the acute study of clinical effectiveness of nesiritide in decompensated heart failure trial (ASCEND-HF). Am Heart J 2009;157(2):271–7.

19. O'Connor CM, Starling RC, Hernandez AF, et al. Effect of nesiritide in patients with acute decompensated heart failure. N Engl J Med 2011;365(1):32–43.

20. Collins SP, Levy PD, Pang PS, et al. The role of the emergency department in acute heart failure clinical trials: enriching patient identification and enrollment. Am Heart J 2013;165(6):902–9.

21. Weintraub NL, Collins SP, Pang PS, et al. Acute heart failure syndromes: emergency department presentation, treatment, and disposition: current approaches and future aims. A scientific statement from the American Heart Association. Circulation 2010;122(19):1975–96.

22. Peacock WF, Braunwald E, Abraham W, et al. National Heart, Lung, and Blood Institute working group on emergency department management of acute heart failure: research challenges and opportunities. J Am Coll Cardiol 2010;56(5):343–51.

23. Peacock WF, Chandra A, Char D, et al. Clevidipine in acute heart failure: results of the A Study of Blood Pressure Control in Acute Heart Failure-A Pilot Study (PRONTO). Am Heart J 2014;167(4):529–36.

24. Whellan DJ, Kraus WE, Kitzman DW, et al. Authorship in a multicenter clinical trial: the Heart Failure-A Controlled Trial Investigating Outcomes of Exercise Training (HF-ACTION) Authorship and Publication (HAP) scoring system results. Am Heart J 2015;169(4):457–63.e6.

Hospitalized Heart Failure in the United States

Lessons Learned from Clinical Trial Populations

Stephen J. Greene, MD[a],*, Lora AlKhawam, MD[b],
Andrew P. Ambrosy, MD[a], Muthiah Vaduganathan, MD, MPH[c],
Robert J. Mentz, MD[a,d]

KEYWORDS

- Heart failure • Clinical trials • North America • Hospitalization

KEY POINTS

- Patients from the United States (US) constitute a minority of those included in prior hospitalized heart failure (HHF) trials.
- The clinical profile, therapy utilization, and postdischarge outcomes of North American HHF trial patients differ from patients enrolled in other areas of the world, although in inconsistent ways.
- Poor enrollment and differing patient characteristics from North America may influence the success of multinational HHF trials and limit the generalizability of results to US patients.
- The continued execution of global HHF trials with the previously documented degree of regional heterogeneity should be re-evaluated. Utilization of a pretrial registry or region-specific trials may be considered.

In the United States (US) alone, the current prevalence of heart failure (HF) is nearly 6 million cases, and this is expected to exceed 8 million cases by 2030 (ie, 1 in every 33 Americans).[1,2] Frequent hospitalization represents the major cause of morbidity for these patients and much of the current understanding of hospitalized HF (HHF) comes from large registry databases.[3–5] However, the primary focus of these American registries has been on the inpatient period, with scant and inconsistent assessment of postdischarge outcomes (excluding linkage to administrative databases). In addition, these registries often include more modest data capture and lack the rigorous and serial measurement of clinical and laboratory parameters and adjudicated outcomes typical of

Funding: None.
Disclosures: R.J. Mentz receives research support from Amgen, AstraZeneca, Bristol-Myers Squibb, GlaxoSmithKline, Gilead, Novartis, Otsuka, and ResMed; honoraria from Thoratec; and has served on an advisory board for Luitpold Pharmaceuticals, Inc. All other authors report no conflicts.
[a] Division of Cardiology, Department of Medicine, Duke University Medical Center, 2301 Erwin Road, Durham, NC 27705, USA; [b] Department of Emergency Medicine, Northwestern University Feinberg School of Medicine, 211 East Ontario Street, Chicago, IL 60611, USA; [c] Heart & Vascular Center, Brigham and Women's Hospital, 75 Francis Street, Boston, MA, USA; [d] Duke Clinical Research Institute, 2400 Pratt Street, Durham, NC 27705, USA
* Corresponding author. Division of Cardiology, Department of Medicine, Duke University Medical Center, 2301 Erwin Road, Suite 7400, Durham, NC 27705, USA.
E-mail address: stephen.greene@dm.duke.edu

Heart Failure Clin 11 (2015) 591–601
http://dx.doi.org/10.1016/j.hfc.2015.07.003
1551-7136/15/$ – see front matter © 2015 Elsevier Inc. All rights reserved.

contemporary clinical trials. Thus, although subject to their own set of limitations, close examination of trial data from North America offers opportunity for incremental granular perspectives on longitudinal HHF patient profiles, care practices, and clinical outcomes in the context of other global populations. With increasing attention being paid to geographic heterogeneity in recent multinational phase 3 HHF trials and its potential influence on study results and generalizability, special focus on the North American subgroup is warranted to inform US regulators, guideline writers, payers, and clinicians.[6,7] Moreover, as most recent HHF clinical trials have failed to identify novel therapies that improve postdischarge outcomes, reflection on the marked regional variation seen in past studies and the participation of US centers will be important for optimizing future drug development programs. The purpose of this article is to describe the available HHF clinical trial data from North America, contextualize the role of these data for improving clinical trial design and conduct in HHF, and discuss potential solutions for improving North American enrollment and ensuring study results are generalizable to US patients.

UNITED STATES STUDY ENROLLMENT

Among the most discussed facets of US clinical trial conduct are the difficulties in enrolling patients and the generally low trial representation compared with other areas of the world.[8–10] Indeed, only 5% of acute care hospitals in the United States routinely participate in clinical trials, necessitating robust enrollment from abroad in order to generate adequate sample sizes.[11] US enrollment in HHF trials is no exception, with the most recently completed trial including only 8% of patients from North America.[12] Review of the 5 most recent HHF trials shows 3 of the 5 trials had North American enrollment rates of no more than 15% (**Table 1**).

The poor recruitment from US centers presents multiple obstacles for completing a well-executed study and for meaningful interpretation of results (**Table 2**). At the forefront is the issue of generalizability to North American patients. Whether secondary to geographic differences in patient level factors (eg, HF pathophysiology, lifestyle, or comorbidities), care practices (eg, therapy utilization, physician reimbursement, medical/legal liability, or threshold for hospitalization/discharge) or local trial site factors (eg, interpretation of selection criteria, enrollment rate, protocol adherence, data collection, and accuracy), patients enrolled within recent HHF trials differ markedly by geographic region.[7,13–15] Comparatively modest US enrollment amplifies these potential influences and increases uncertainty regarding applicability of data to North America. In addition, shifting the burden of patient enrollment abroad carries the risk of relying on foreign sites, where data accuracy and quality control may be in question.[8] Although not a trial of hospitalized, but rather ambulatory HF patients, the recent TOPCAT (Treatment of Preserved Cardiac Function Heart Failure with an Aldosterone Antagonist) trial is one noteworthy example. Within the study, placebo event rates from Russia and the Republic of Georgia were more than 3 times lower than those in other countries, prompting skepticism as

Table 1
North American enrollment in recent hospitalized heart failure trials

Trial	Year Published	Protocol Specified Time from Admission to Randomization	Total Enrollment	North American Enrollment	% Enrolled in North American Sites
EVEREST[22]	2007	≤48 h	4133	1251	30%
PROTECT[32]	2010	≤24 h	2033	313	15%
ASCEND-HF[33]	2011	<24 h[a]	7007	3149	45%
RELAX-AHF[34]	2013	≤16 h	1161	114	10%
ASTRONAUT[12]	2013	5 d[b]	1615	124	8%
TOTAL	—	—	15,949	4951	31%

[a] ASCEND-HF protocol allowed either randomization within 24 hours of heart failure admission or within 48 hours of a diagnosis of acute HF after hospitalization for another cause.
[b] ASTRONAUT protocol did not specify a mandatory window within which patients needed to be randomized. Results showed that patients in the trial were randomized a median 5 days after admission overall, and a median 2 days after admission in North America.
  Adapted from Harinstein ME, Butler J, Greene SJ, et al. Site selection for heart failure clinical trials in the USA. Heart Fail Rev 2015;20(4):377; with permission.

Table 2
Concerns about conducting clinical trials outside the United States

Variant Characteristic	Concern
Patient risk profile	Patient population is not representative
Availability of therapeutic interventions	Proven therapies not always provided
Affordability of therapeutic interventions	—
Availability of hospital infrastructure	—
Availability of clinic infrastructure	Appropriate follow-up and evaluation not provided
Clinical practice and standard of care	Disease progress is not representative
Disease outcomes	Disease epidemiology is not representative
Genetic profile	Effectiveness of therapies is not representative
Cultural/social background	Acceptance of therapies is not representative

Adapted from Butler J, Fonarow GC, O'Connor C, et al. Improving cardiovascular clinical trials conduct in the United States: recommendation from clinicians, researchers, sponsors, and regulators. Am Heart J 2015;169(3):306; with permission.

to the quality of data for nearly half of the overall trial population.[16] Moreover, there was differential efficacy of study drug by region, with spironolactone meeting the primary endpoint in the Americas but failing to do so in the lower-risk cohort from Russia and Republic of Georgia.[16] These findings generated the hypothesis that regional variation in patient profiles, interpretation of trial selection criteria, and/or study execution can strongly influence trial results.[7]

Further complicating poor US participation may be the association between individual site enrollment and patient outcomes. A post hoc analysis from the EVEREST (Efficacy of Vasopressin Antagonism in Heart Failure: Outcome Study with Tolvaptan) trial found patients from sites that enrolled no more than 30 patients had greater risk of cardiovascular mortality or HHF (CVM/HHF).[17] This hazard was further accentuated in the 25% of sites enrolling no more than 10 patients. Although the influence of site enrollment on outcome did not differ by geographic region,

a notable 75% of sites in the lowest enrolling group were from North America. Overall, North American sites enrolled an average of only 7.2 patients over the course of the trial. This relationship between site enrollment and clinical outcomes has yet to be validated in another HHF cohort, but nonetheless suggests that despite strict patient selection criteria, the site enrollment rate may bias results. Thus, from the North American perspective, poor site enrollment rate may further compound other consequences from poor national representation on study applicability.

PATIENT CHARACTERISTICS

The demographic, vital sign, and comorbidity burden of North Americans enrolled in 4 multinational HHF trials with available regional data are displayed **Table 3**.[13–15,18] Approximately 50% of patients had a history of diabetes and approximately 80% to 90% had a history of hypertension. Patient ages ranged from 59 to 67 years, and nearly three-quarters of the North American populations were men. North Americans tended to have the highest baseline weights (87–98.5 kg) and the lowest baseline ejection fractions ($\sim$25%) among all patients in the trials. In general, rates of coronary revascularization were highest in North America and differed markedly from multiple other regions, particularly Eastern Europe and Russia. For instance, in PROTECT (Placebo-Controlled Randomized Study of the Selective A1 Adenosine Receptor Antagonist Rolofylline for Patients Hospitalized with Acute Decompensated Heart Failure and Volume Overload to Assess Treatment Effect on Congestion and Renal Function), rates of prior percutaneous coronary intervention and coronary bypass grafting in Russia were 1% and 2%, respectively, compared with 26% and 38% in North America. This discrepancy was seen despite patients enrolled from Russia having a substantially higher rate of prior myocardial infarction (60% vs 41%). For the purposes of planning future multinational HHF trials, potential regional underutilization of revascularization for coronary artery disease may carry significant implications, as angina and HF can present with similar symptoms (eg, dyspnea). This could be especially problematic in HFpEF trials in which the initial HF diagnosis may be more challenging. It is notable that in TOPCAT, patients from the Republic of Georgia and Russia also had significantly lower rates of prior revascularization and higher rates of baseline angina as compared with the Americas.[19]

Data from these trials also suggest that North Americans have the highest N-terminal pro-B-type natriuretic peptide (NT-proBNP) levels near

Table 3
Baseline characteristics of North American patients enrolled in global hospitalized heart failure trials

	EVEREST	PROTECT	ASCEND-HF[a]	ASTRONAUT
Enrollment data				
Number of patients	1251 (30.3)	313 (15.4)	2684 (38.3)	123 (7.6)
Number of sites	173 (48.2)	—	—	43 (14.9)
Number of patients per site	7.2	—	—	2.9 ± 2.4
Demographics				
Age (y)	67.5 ± 12.8	67 (57–77)	67 (55–78)	59.2 ± 13.5
Male (%)	74.7	74	64.5	75.6
Race (%)				
Caucasian	75.4	71	60.5	46.3
Black	18.5	—	—	50.4
Other	6.2	—	—	3.2
Time from admission to randomization (d)	—	—	—	2 (2–4)
Hospital length of stay (d)	4 (3–7)	5 (4–8)	5 (4–8)	5 (3–7)
Ejection fraction (%)	24.6 ± 8.5	25.0 (20.0–35.0)[b]	71.8% with EF <40%	23.6 ± 7.8
Ischemic HF etiology (%)	—	63	—	48.4
NYHA class at baseline (%)				
I/II	—	—	—	25.2
III/IV	95.7	—	—	73.2
Missing	4.3	—	—	1.6
Atrial fibrillation on baseline electrocardiogram (ECG) (%)	15.5	—	—	17.0
QRS duration on baseline ECG (ms)	—	—	—	122 ± 34
QRS ≥120 ms (%)	42.2[c]	—	—	—
Vital sign and laboratory data				
Systolic blood pressure (mm Hg)	116.6 ± 19.2	114 (103–131)	125 (111–142)	128.7 ± 18.0
Heart rate (bpm)	78.1 ± 14.6	76 (67–87)	79 (70–90)	82.5 ± 15.1
Weight (kg)	87.5 ± 20.9	87 (74–103)	88 (74–106)	98.5 ± 28.9
Body mass index (kg/m^2)	—	29 (25–35)	—	33.0 ± 9.3
Hemoglobin (g/dL)	—	11.7 (10.6–13.3)	12.3 (11.0–13.7)	13.0 ± 1.9
Serum sodium (mmol/L)	139.9 ± 4.4	138 (135–140)	139 (137–141)	139.9 ± 2.9
Serum potassium (mmol/L)	—	4.0 (3.6–4.4)	—	4.1 ± 0.5
Blood urea nitrogen (mg/dL)	35.1 ± 19.6	33 (23–48)	8.2 (6.1–12.1)	26.1 ± 11.5
Creatinine (mg/dL)	1.5 ± 0.5	1.5 (1.2–2.0)	1.3 (1.0–1.7)	1.2 ± 0.3
eGFR (mL/min/1.73 m^2)	—	43 (31–56)	—	68.3 ± 21.4
NT-proBNP at admission (pg/mL)	—	—	—	5660 (3021–8600)
NT-proBNP at baseline (pg/mL)	—	86% with ≥3000 pg/mL	—	2555 (1395–4900)
BNP at admission (pg/mL)	—	—	—	1110 (650–2038)
BNP at baseline (pg/mL)	1031 (470–2100)	1288 (863–2120)	—	423 (219–871)
Past medical history (%)				
Previous HF hospitalization	80.2	—	—	75.6

(continued on next page)

Table 3
(continued)

	EVEREST	PROTECT	ASCEND-HF[a]	ASTRONAUT
Coronary artery disease	77.4	—	61.5	52.0
Previous PCI	32.6	26	—	29.3
Previous coronary artery bypass grafting	41.4	38	—	23.6
Previous myocardial infarction	55.5	41	34.2	36.6
Previous stroke	—	—	—	12.2
Hypertension	78.7	82	83.5	94.3
Atrial fibrillation	—	49	40.8	34.1
Diabetes	51.6	53	49.1	52.8
Chronic obstructive pulmonary disease	18.1	30	25.6	26.0
Medications at discharge (%)				
Diuretics	93.1	—	90.1	90.2
Beta-blockers	81.8	88	84.5	91.9
ACEI/ARB	77.4	71	70.9	87.0
MRA	42.7	41	33.6	32.5
MRA + ACEI/ARB	—	—	—	26.8
Digoxin	48.8	32	5.9	23.6
ICD	34.2	—	37.7	38.2
CRT	—	—	21.1	11.4
Permanent pacemaker	13.4	—	—	19.5

Data are expressed as mean ± standard deviation, median (interquartile range), or n (%).

Abbreviations: ACEI, angiotensin-converting enzyme inhibitor; ARB, angiotensin II receptor blocker; BNP, B-type natriuretic peptide; CRT, cardiac resynchronization therapy; EF, ejection fraction; eGFR, estimated glomerular filtration rate; HF, heart failure; ICD, implantable cardioverter-defibrillator; MRA, mineralocorticoid receptor antagonist; NT-proBNP, N-terminal pro-B-type natriuretic peptide; NYHA, New York Heart Association; PCI, percutaneous coronary intervention.

[a] Data from ASCEND-HF reflect US patients only. Data from all other trials represent North America patients.
[b] Only 48% of patients in the PROTECT trial had an ejection fraction measurement.
[c] Number of QRS measurements in North America in EVEREST n = 632.

Data from Refs.[13–15,18]

the time of HF admission. In EVEREST, serum B-type natriuretic peptide (BNP) among North Americans was more than 40% greater than the next highest region. In PROTECT, more than 85% of patients from North America had an NT-proBNP level greater than 3000 pg/mL at enrollment, the highest such proportion of any region. Similar findings were seen in ASTRONAUT (Aliskiren Trial on Acute Heart Failure Outcomes). However, data from ASTRONAUT also characterized the in-hospital natriuretic peptide trajectory for these patients. Unlike other HHF trials, randomization in ASTRONAUT did not occur within 24 to 48 hours of initial presentation, but rather occurred a median of 5 days after admission while the patient was still hospitalized. Among North Americans, there was a robust reduction in NT-proBNP level between admission and randomization by greater than 50%. This large decrease in natriuretic peptide level occurred despite North American

patients having the shortest time from admission to enrollment (ie, median 2 days) of any region. By contrast, in Eastern Europe, NT-proBNP decreased only marginally from median 3000 pg/mL to 2537 pg/mL despite the region having the longest duration between presentation and enrollment (ie, median 6 days). With the caveat being that admission and randomization levels were drawn at local and core laboratories, respectively, the rapid improvement in NT-proBNP in North America in ASTRONAUT may speak to a selectively low risk profile or heightened intensity of standard in-hospital therapy in this region.

In contrast, other North American characteristics differed markedly across HHF trials. For example, North Americans in EVEREST and PROTECT had the lowest systolic blood pressures in the trial (mean 116.6 mm Hg and median 114 mm Hg, respectively), whereas they had by far the highest in ASTRONAUT (mean 128.7 mm Hg). The percentage of North Americans identified as black ranged from 18.5% in EVEREST to 50.4% in ASTRONAUT. Rates of prior myocardial infarction ranged from 34.2 in ASCEND-HF (Acute Study of Clinical Effectiveness of Nesiritide in Decompensated Heart Failure) to 55.5% in EVEREST. Thus, specific study entry criteria may further influence the selection of patient populations and further accentuate regional differences.

LENGTH OF STAY AND READMISSION RISK

Data exploring the association between length of stay (LOS) and rehospitalization risk among HHF patients are limited, but recent analyses from HHF trial databases offer insights into the complex relationship. In the ASCEND-HF (Acute Study of Clinical Effectiveness of Nesiritide in Decompensated Heart Failure) database, Eapen and colleagues[20] demonstrated an inverse relationship between country-level mean LOS and readmission risk, with each additional hospital day across countries independently associated with a 14% and 21% lower risk of 30-day all-cause and HF readmission, respectively. Specifically, data from the United States showed a mean LOS of 6.1 days and a 17.8% 30-day all-cause readmission rate. More recently, Khan and colleagues[21] published data from EVEREST assessing LOS implications with incremental insights related to cause-specific readmissions (eg, all-cause, HF, cardiovascular non-HF, and noncardiovascular hospitalization). Similar to the ASCEND-HF study, increased LOS was independently associated with lower risk of 30-day HF readmissions in the overall EVEREST cohort. However, in a region-specific analysis within North America, this relationship became nonsignificant. Moreover, and in contrast with the ASCEND-HF analysis, increased LOS independently predicted heightened risk of all-cause readmission, both in the overall EVEREST cohort and among North Americans. These same relationships were also statistically significant for cardiovascular non-HF readmissions, while trends existed for increased risk of noncardiovascular readmission. Among North Americans included in EVEREST, the median LOS was 4 days, and the 30-day all-cause readmission rate was 23.5%.

Khan and colleagues[21] commented on potential reasons for the discordant results from these 2 trial datasets. They noted similar 30-day HF readmission rates of 5.4% to 5.6% between the 2 studies, yet a substantially higher all-cause readmission rate in EVEREST, and suggest that differing comorbidity burdens and risks of non-HF rehospitalization may explain the findings in EVEREST. Furthermore, differing definitions of the 30-day

period (ie, 30-days after randomization in ASCEND-HF vs 30-days after discharge in EVEREST) and associated differences in at-risk readmission time may have influenced results. Lastly, while the ASCEND-HF analysis utilized a continuous variable technique to calculate incremental risk per additional hospital day, Khan and colleagues categorized LOS by quintile. It is notable that all statistically significant results in the EVEREST analysis occurred by comparing quintile 5 ($\geq$14 days) with quintile 1 ($\leq$3 days). Although there were some trends toward a graded relationship, intermediate LOS quintiles did not carry independent predictive value.

Based on the previously described data, the exact nature of the relationship between LOS and rehospitalization risk remains unclear. Efforts to better understand this correlation are complicated by multiple confounders that may influence readmissions and are not specific to HF, including transitions of care and postdischarge follow-up procedures, physician reimbursement, medical-legal liability, and patient expectations. As the 30-day readmission rate continues to be a quality-of-care measure, further comprehensive research and quality improvement efforts to reduce hospitalizations are needed, with LOS representing only 1 component of the risk assessment for individual patients.

THERAPY UTILIZATION

In HHF trials, baseline treatment with angiotensin-converting enzyme inhibitors (ACEIs)/angiotensin II receptor blockers (ARBs) and beta-blocker therapy in North America is generally greater than 70%, with beta-blocker use consistently the highest among all regions. By comparison, use of mineralocorticoid receptor antagonists (MRAs) and digoxin is consistently near the lowest. Data are also available regarding in-hospital initiation and discontinuation of medications. In PROTECT, the net incremental uptake of ACEIs/ARBs, beta-blockers, and MRAs were +2%, +4%, and +7%, respectively.[14] Similar findings were seen in EVEREST, while in-hospital addition of therapy was more robust in ASCEND-HF (ie, $\geq$9% for all 3 drugs).[13,18] Despite these data being derived from clinical trials where patients receive rigorous protocol prespecified follow-up, the use of guideline therapies in these databases is similar to that seen among reduced ejection fraction patients from recent North American registries.[5]

Overall, utilization of evidence-based device therapy continues to be low in HHF trials. Despite all patients enrolled in EVEREST and ASTRONAUT having reduced EF and a history of chronic HF, only approximately 15% of patients had an implantable cardioverter–defibrillator (ICD).[12,22] Although the prevalence was highest in North America, ICD rates still fell below 40%, much lower than the rate of 54% seen in North America in the recent PARADIGM-HF (Prospective Comparison of ARNI with ACEI to Determine Impact on Global Mortality and Morbidity in Heart Failure) trial of chronic ambulatory patients.[13,15,23] Use of cardiac resynchronization therapy in ASTRONAUT was similarly low in North America (11.4%), but was higher than all other regions except Western Europe.

In summary, North Americans show a relatively consistent pattern in use of background therapies across recent HHF trials. However, utilization of many treatments differs markedly from other global regions and may contribute to differences in event rates and modes of death.

CLINICAL OUTCOMES

Among the global regional analyses from EVEREST, PROTECT, and ASTRONAUT, the worldwide variation in clinical outcomes has likely received the most attention. Blair and colleagues[13] first documented this heterogeneity in EVEREST, in which even after adjustment for patient characteristics and therapies, South Americans carried an increased risk of death, and Eastern Europeans carried an increased risk of CVM/HHF, relative to North Americans. Global heterogeneity was also

documented in PROTECT, in which, compared with Western Europe, patients from Eastern Europe and Russia experienced significantly lower 60-day rehospitalization risk, and patients from North America and Israel carried lower 60-day mortality risk. Most recently, the ASTRONAUT investigators published a striking example of regional variation in outcomes among HHF patients.[15] Despite adjustment for baseline patient characteristics, relative to North America, enrollment in Latin America and Eastern Europe was associated with a greater than 2-fold increased risk of death. The risk was greater than 3 fold greater in the Asia/Pacific region.

Although the previously mentioned regional analyses repeatedly document marked global differences in outcomes, the findings from North America are not consistent (**Fig. 1**). This becomes more apparent when one considers the raw events rates from North America within the trials. For example, in EVEREST, the estimated 1-year rates of mortality and CVM/HHF in North America were the highest of any region at 30.4% and 52.5%, respectively. The North American mortality rate was similarly high in PROTECT, measuring 20.1% at 6 months. In sharp contrast, although rates of 1 year CVM/HHF in ASTRONAUT were again highest in North America (47.2%), the 1-year mortality rate was exceedingly low at 7.3%, less than half that of any other region and rivaling mortality rates seen in other recent ambulatory chronic HFrEF trials.[24,25]

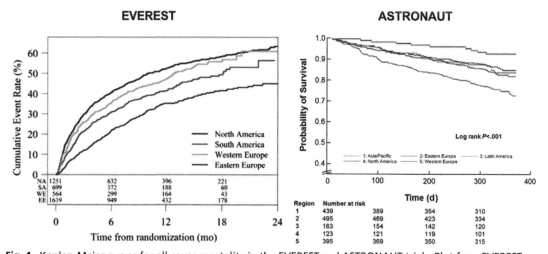

Fig. 1. Kaplan-Meier curves for all-cause mortality in the EVEREST and ASTRONAUT trials. Plot from EVEREST represents event rates over the duration of trial follow-up (median 9.9 months). Plot from ASTRONAUT represents probability of survival up to 1 year after randomization. (*Adapted from* Blair JE, Zannad F, Konstam MA, et al. Continental differences in clinical characteristics, management, and outcomes in patients hospitalized with worsening heart failure results from the EVEREST (Efficacy of Vasopressin Antagonism in Heart Failure: outcome Study with Tolvaptan) program. J Am Coll Cardiol 2008;52(20):1644; and Greene SJ, Fonarow GC, Solomon SD, et al. Global variation in clinical profile, management, and post-discharge outcomes among patients hospitalized for worsening chronic heart failure: findings from the ASTRONAUT trial. Eur J Heart Fail 2015;17(6):598.)

Explanations for the remarkably few North American deaths in ASTRONAUT may be related to the baseline patient characteristics, the rapid and sizable reduction of in-hospital NT-proBNP level, increased ICD utilization, and the higher baseline systolic blood pressure. Although these factors were accounted for in multivariable analyses, it is possible that unmeasured factors tracking with these characteristics yielded a lower-risk cohort. Along these lines, perhaps the lack of a prespecified time point for randomization in ASTRONAUT allowed for further differentiation of risk profiles during the hospitalization, with North American investigators selectively enrolling patients with a favorable in-hospital course. The low enrollment rate of 2.9 patients per site in North America suggests a highly selected cohort. A second hypothesis relates to a varying threshold for hospitalization across world regions. A low threshold for hospitalization in North America could foster inclusion of patients with low biologic HF risk, as evidenced by low risk of death (ie, an objective biologic endpoint) but paradoxically high risk of recurrent HHF (as evidenced by the index admission). Regardless of mechanism, the low North American mortality rate seen in ASTRONAUT is clearly an outlier in the HHF literature. However, it provides a startling reminder on how interpretation and implementation of a clinical trial protocol can differ by geographic region and limit generalizability of results.

POTENTIAL FUTURE DIRECTIONS FOR UNITED STATES TRIALS

It is unclear whether continued execution of HHF trials with the previously reported degree of global heterogeneity is worthwhile and reasonably capable of bringing efficacious therapies to clinical practice. Marked regional variation within a trial conflicts strongly with the US Food and Drug Administration mandate that data from international trials be relevant to US medical practice.[8] Moreover, heterogeneity and differing treatment effects set the stage for 3 potentially problematic scenarios[26]:

1. The overall trial endpoint is met, but a specific region derives no benefit or harm.
2. The overall trial endpoint is not met because of offsetting benefits and harms in different regions, and a potentially useful therapy is abandoned.
3. The overall trial endpoint is met, but because of global heterogeneity, the size of the effect is small, and despite meeting regulatory approval, the therapy is not widely accepted by clinicians and/or payers.

Potential solutions to reduce global variation in HHF trials and maximize generalizability to the United States are presented in **Table 4**. The first potential solution is a pretrial registry. The goal of such a registry would be to serve as a trial run for study sites prior to potential inclusion in the subsequent clinical trial.[27] Trial leadership and sponsors would be able to evaluate a site's ability to enroll adequate numbers of representative patients, adhere to the registry protocol, perform follow-up, and communicate with the Steering Committee.[27] Although the upfront resources required for a pretrial program would be substantial, the expenses may be modest when one considers the costs of supporting poorly performing sites through the trial duration and the overall costs of unsuccessful phase 3 programs. For purposes of reducing global heterogeneity, a pretrial registry could provide quality control, ensuring that characteristics and patient outcomes across sites during the registry period are roughly similar and consistent with the targeted risk profile. Sites associated with suspiciously divergent patient profiles or outcomes could be scrutinized with potential exclusion from the subsequent phase 3 study.

A second, and perhaps more radical, proposal is to limit specific trials to the United States or North America only. Although this approach deviates from the more conventional belief that phase 3 trials should be designed to include developing countries, focusing enrollment to specific areas of the world may be the most failsafe way of ensuring applicability to a given population.[10,28] For the purposes of a trial limited to North America, critics may point to problems with cost containment and slow enrollment rates as hurdles. However, executing such a trial in conjunction with a US pretrial registry may be the ideal means of identifying high-performing sites capable of meeting enrollment requirements.[8] Moreover, combined execution with a registry could allow a trial to leverage pre-existing registry infrastructure. For example, 2 registry-based percutaneous coronary intervention trials successfully utilized electronic health records and registry systems already in place to efficiently conduct large-scale trials.[29,30] Likewise, the recently initiated ADAPT-ABLE (Aspirin Dosing: A Patient-centric Trial Assessing Benefits and Long-term Effectiveness) study, the first approved pragmatic study under direction of the US PCORnet (Patient-Centered Clinical Research Network) program, plans to include only US sites and to utilize existing electronic health records and Web-based patient portals to enroll and follow 20,000 patients. Similar approaches could be considered in the HHF trial

Table 4
Potential strategies for improving generalizability of hospitalized heart failure trial results to US patients

Strategy	Advantages or Examples
Pretrial registry	• Ensure appropriateness of patient characteristics and clinical outcomes associated with potential study sites • Provides a trial run to better judge a site's ability to follow a study protocol, accurately collect data, and provide postdischarge follow-up • Use site event rates to better estimate enrollment required for adequate statistical power • Ensure adequate site compliance with current standards of care • Partially trains the centers for potential inclusion in subsequent trials
Trials limited to specific geographic regions (eg, United States, North America)	• Improve generalizability of trial results to a specific global region • Selectively test investigational therapies with unclear risk/benefit in countries that might realistically be able to access them in a timely manner should they be approved
Improve US enrollment	• Pragmatic trials with easier eligibility criteria and streamlined protocols • Combine trial enrollment/follow-up with routine care or an ongoing registry via the electronic health record • Better incentivize local investigators and hospitals to participate in clinical trials • Develop regional research networks with independent staff dedicated to conducting trials across a group of affiliated hospitals • Raise public and physician awareness regarding the scope of the hospitalized heart failure problem • Include clinical trials training within residencies and fellowships and facilitate participation in clinical events committees and data safety monitoring boards • Prespecify trial enrollment quotas for each geographic region

space to bolster enrollment and make a trial limited to the United States feasible.

An additional rationale for a trial limited to North America relates to the current pharmaceutical climate and the high initial cost of newly approved therapies. Although study sponsors may find less-developed countries appealing for clinical trials from a regulatory and cost standpoint, these areas are paradoxically more likely to find newly approved drugs prohibitively expensive, and routine utilization may only occur after years of use in wealthier countries. Ethical questions exist regarding testing investigational therapies with uncertain risks/benefits in less-developed countries if those populations will not be able to reasonably afford them in a timely manner should they be approved. Although less-developed countries often enroll a substantial percentage of trial cohorts, patients from developed global regions may be disproportionately more likely to reap the early postapproval downstream benefits of efficacious new treatments.

In summary, a pragmatic approach going forward may be to test therapies in a more homogeneous cohort within North America or another specified geographic location. Such a strategy

may maximize likelihood of improving outcomes for the specified patient subset. Moreover, this approach could set the stage for the therapy to be serially trialed in other global regions to assess for generalizability of effect and potentially allow time for the costs of therapy to fall and global access to improve.[31] Concurrent use of a pretrial registry to identify high-performing sites for study inclusion could obviate concerns over poor North American enrollment rates. On the other hand, if global trials are to continue, at the very least, it seems appropriate to mandate prespecified regional analyses and regional enrollment quotas to allow meaningful regional interaction analyses.

SUMMARY

Randomized controlled trials continue to be the cornerstone of evidence-based medicine and will undoubtedly be the avenue by which future life-saving therapies for HHF are discovered. North American patients have made up a minority of those included in these studies and have been shown to consistently differ from patients from other areas of the world, although in inconsistent ways. Unless methods to account for this global variation are implemented, these differences raise concerns over applicability of future trial results to the United States and present a significant hurdle for regulatory agency approval should a successful overall trial result be achieved. Thus, recognizing the varying patient profiles and outcomes of North Americans enrolled in prior HHF trial programs is critical to optimizing design of future drug development programs and maximizing chances of bringing a novel therapeutic agent to the bedside.

REFERENCES

1. Go AS, Mozaffarian D, Roger VL, et al. Heart disease and stroke statistics–2014 update: a report from the American Heart Association. Circulation 2014;129(3):e28–292.

2. Heidenreich PA, Albert NM, Allen LA, et al. Forecasting the impact of heart failure in the United States: a policy statement from the American Heart Association. Circ Heart Fail 2013;6(3):606–19.

3. Gheorghiade M, Abraham WT, Albert NM, et al. Systolic blood pressure at admission, clinical characteristics, and outcomes in patients hospitalized with acute heart failure. JAMA 2006;296(18):2217–26.

4. Adams KF Jr, Fonarow GC, Emerman CL, et al. Characteristics and outcomes of patients hospitalized for heart failure in the United States: rationale, design, and preliminary observations from the first 100,000 cases in the Acute Decompensated Heart Failure National Registry (ADHERE). Am Heart J 2005;149(2):209–16.

5. Steinberg BA, Zhao X, Heidenreich PA, et al. Trends in patients hospitalized with heart failure and preserved left ventricular ejection fraction: prevalence, therapies, and outcomes. Circulation 2012;126(1): 65–75.

6. Mentz RJ, Kaski JC, Dan GA, et al. Implications of geographical variation on clinical outcomes of cardiovascular trials. Am Heart J 2012;164(3):303–12.

7. Pitt B, Gheorghiade M. Geographic variation in heart failure trials: time for scepticism? Eur J Heart Fail 2014;16(6):601–2.

8. Harinstein ME, Butler J, Greene SJ, et al. Site selection for heart failure clinical trials in the USA. Heart Fail Rev 2015;20(4):375–83.

9. Gheorghiade M, Vaduganathan M, Greene SJ, et al. Site selection in global clinical trials in patients hospitalized for heart failure: perceived problems and potential solutions. Heart Fail Rev 2014;19(2): 135–52.

10. Butler J, Fonarow GC, O'Connor C, et al. Improving cardiovascular clinical trials conduct in the United States: recommendation from clinicians, researchers, sponsors, and regulators. Am Heart J 2015;169(3): 305–14.

11. Califf RM, Harrington RA. American industry and the U.S. cardiovascular clinical research enterprise an appropriate analogy? J Am Coll Cardiol 2011; 58(7):677–80.

12. Gheorghiade M, Bohm M, Greene SJ, et al. Effect of aliskiren on postdischarge mortality and heart failure readmissions among patients hospitalized for heart failure: the ASTRONAUT randomized trial. JAMA 2013;309(11):1125–35.

13. Blair JE, Zannad F, Konstam MA, et al. Continental differences in clinical characteristics, management, and outcomes in patients hospitalized with worsening heart failure results from the EVEREST (Efficacy of Vasopressin Antagonism in Heart Failure: outcome Study with Tolvaptan) program. J Am Coll Cardiol 2008;52(20):1640–8.

14. Mentz RJ, Cotter G, Cleland JG, et al. International differences in clinical characteristics, management, and outcomes in acute heart failure patients: better short-term outcomes in patients enrolled in Eastern Europe and Russia in the PROTECT trial. Eur J Heart Fail 2014;16(6):614–24.

15. Greene SJ, Fonarow GC, Solomon SD, et al. Global variation in clinical profile, management, and postdischarge outcomes among patients hospitalized for worsening chronic heart failure: findings from the ASTRONAUT trial. Eur J Heart Fail 2015;17(6): 591–600.

16. Pitt B, Pfeffer MA, Assmann SF, et al. Spironolactone for heart failure with preserved ejection fraction. N Engl J Med 2014;370(15):1383–92.

17. Butler J, Subacius H, Vaduganathan M, et al. Relationship between clinical trial site enrollment with participant characteristics, protocol completion, and outcomes: insights from the EVEREST (Efficacy of Vasopressin Antagonism in Heart Failure: outcome Study with Tolvaptan) trial. J Am Coll Cardiol 2013;61(5):571–9.

18. Kaul P, Reed SD, Hernandez AF, et al. Differences in treatment, outcomes, and quality of life among patients with heart failure in Canada and the United States. JACC Heart Fail 2013;1(6):523–30.

19. Pfeffer MA, Claggett B, Assmann SF, et al. regional variation in patients and outcomes in the Treatment of Preserved Cardiac Function Heart Failure With an Aldosterone Antagonist (TOPCAT) Trial. Circulation 2015;131(1):34–42.

20. Eapen ZJ, Reed SD, Li Y, et al. Do countries or hospitals with longer hospital stays for acute heart failure have lower readmission rates?: findings from ASCEND-HF. Circ Heart Fail 2013;6(4):727–32.

21. Khan H, Greene SJ, Fonarow GC, et al. Length of hospital stay and 30-day readmission following heart failure hospitalization: insights from the EVEREST trial. Eur J Heart Fail 2015. [Epub ahead of print].

22. Konstam MA, Gheorghiade M, Burnett JC Jr, et al. Effects of oral tolvaptan in patients hospitalized for

worsening heart failure: the EVEREST Outcome Trial. JAMA 2007;297(12):1319–31.

23. McMurray JJ, Packer M, Solomon SD. Neprilysin inhibition for heart failure. N Engl J Med 2014;371(24): 2336–7.

24. Swedberg K, Komajda M, Bohm M, et al. Ivabradine and outcomes in chronic heart failure (SHIFT): a randomised placebo-controlled study. Lancet 2010;376(9744):875–85.

25. McMurray JJ, Packer M, Desai AS, et al. Angiotensin-neprilysin inhibition versus enalapril in heart failure. N Engl J Med 2014;371(11):993–1004.

26. Greene SJ, Gheorghiade M. Reply: considerations for drug development for heart failure. J Am Coll Cardiol 2015;65(10):1061–2.

27. Greene SJ, Shah AN, Butler J, et al. Designing effective drug and device development programs for hospitalized heart failure: a proposal for pretrial registries. Am Heart J 2014;168(2):142–9.

28. Stough WG, Zannad F, Pitt B, et al. Globalization of cardiovascular clinical research: the balance between meeting medical needs and maintaining scientific standards. Am Heart J 2007;154(2):232–8.

29. Hess CN, Rao SV, Kong DF, et al. Embedding a randomized clinical trial into an ongoing registry infrastructure: unique opportunities for efficiency in design of the Study of Access site For Enhancement of Percutaneous Coronary Intervention for Women (SAFE-PCI for Women). Am Heart J 2013;166(3):421–8.

30. Frobert O, Lagerqvist B, Olivecrona GK, et al. Thrombus aspiration during ST-segment elevation myocardial infarction. N Engl J Med 2013;369(17): 1587–97.

31. Greene SJ, Gheorghiade M. Matching mechanism of death with mechanism of action: considerations for drug development for hospitalized heart failure. J Am Coll Cardiol 2014;64(15):1599–601.

32. Massie BM, O'Connor CM, Metra M, et al. Rolofylline, an adenosine A1-receptor antagonist, in acute heart failure. N Engl J Med 2010;363(15):1419–28.

33. O'Connor CM, Starling RC, Hernandez AF, et al. Effect of nesiritide in patients with acute decompensated heart failure. N Engl J Med 2011;365(1):32–43.

34. Teerlink JR, Cotter G, Davison BA, et al. Serelaxin, recombinant human relaxin-2, for treatment of acute heart failure (RELAX-AHF): a randomised, placebo-controlled trial. Lancet 2013;381(9860):29–39.

The Impact of Worsening Heart Failure in the United States

Lauren B. Cooper, MD*, Adam D. DeVore, MD,
G. Michael Felker, MD, MHS

KEYWORDS

- Worsening heart failure • Clinical trials • Outcomes • Medications

KEY POINTS

- In-hospital worsening heart failure is an increasingly important endpoint in trials of acute heart failure.
- In-hospital worsening heart failure is associated with increased short- and long-term mortality, rehospitalization, and health care costs.
- Renal dysfunction and cardiac dysfunction predict worsening heart failure in patients hospitalized with acute heart failure.
- A standardized definition of worsening heart failure should be established for use in future clinical trials.

INTRODUCTION AND DEFINITIONS

Heart failure is a common condition in the United States. More than 5 million Americans have heart failure, with more than 800,000 new cases diagnosed annually.[1] This chronic condition is marked by episodes of acute decompensation, often requiring hospitalization. In the United States alone, there are greater than 1 million hospitalizations annually for acute heart failure.[1] Unfortunately, patient outcomes remain poor with a 5-year survival rate of approximately 50% and there is an urgent public health need to improve our understanding and treatment options for patients suffering with acute heart failure.[1] Acute heart failure therapeutics remain largely homogenous and unchanged over the past 40 years in the United States.[2,3]

The term "worsening heart failure" has been used to indicate worsening of chronic heart failure, also termed "acute heart failure" or "acute decompensated heart failure." This acute worsening of chronic heart failure often results in adjustment of chronic therapy or requires in-patient hospitalization and is associated with worse prognosis.[4,5] Worsening heart failure has also been used to

Disclosures: Dr L.B. Cooper reports receiving research support from Novartis. Dr A.D. DeVore reports receiving research support from Amgen, the American Heart Association, Novartis, Maquet, and Thoratec, and serving as a consultant for Maquet. Dr G.M. Felker reports receiving grant support from the National Heart, Lung, and Blood Institute, Novartis, Roche Diagnostics, Otsuka, and Amgen, and serving as a consulting for Trevena, Amgen, Novartis, Celladon, Sorbent, Bristol-Myers Squibb, Singlulex, St. Jude Medical, and Medtronic.
Funding Source: Dr L.B. Cooper was supported by grant T32HL069749-11A1 from the National Institutes of Health.
Disclaimer: The content is solely the responsibility of the authors and does not necessarily represent the official views of the National Heart, Lung, and Blood Institute, or the National Institutes of Health.
Duke Clinical Research Institute, PO Box 17969, Durham, NC 27715, USA
* Corresponding author.
E-mail address: lauren.b.cooper@duke.edu

heartfailure.theclinics.com

describe worsening of acute heart failure that occurs during a hospitalization for acute heart failure. For the purposes of this review, we focus on the latter condition, namely, in-hospital worsening heart failure.

In-hospital worsening heart failure represents a clinical scenario in which a patient hospitalized for treatment of acute heart failure experiences a worsening of their condition while in the hospital, requiring escalation of therapy. This can occur in patients who do not respond to initial therapy or in those who do respond to initial therapy but subsequently stop responding or worsen. Worsening heart failure can occur at any point throughout the hospitalization.[6,7] There is a growing body of evidence that in-hospital worsening heart failure is also associated with a worse prognosis and signals an important change in the heart failure patient's clinical course (**Fig. 1**). These data suggest therapeutic strategies designed to reduce the incidence of in-hospital worsening heart failure could improve patient outcomes.

ESTABLISHING A DEFINITION FOR WORSENING HEART FAILURE AS A CLINICAL TRIAL ENDPOINT

Several clinical trials in acute heart failure have examined worsening heart failure as an endpoint. The first trial to define and examine worsening heart failure was published in 2004 and compared different doses of tezosentan, an endothelin receptor antagonist with vasodilating properties.[8] This study included patients from centers in Europe, Israel, and the United States. Investigators examined both hemodynamic and clinical endpoints, including worsening heart failure, defined as "either failure to improve (persistent symptoms and signs of acute heart failure during the first 24 h of treatment) or recurrent symptoms and signs of acute heart failure, pulmonary edema, or cardiogenic shock after initial stabilization within 30 days after randomization, either of which required the initiation or increase of appropriate intravenous therapy or the implementation of mechanical circulatory or ventilatory support to treat the event."[8]

The rationale for using worsening heart failure as an endpoint in acute heart failure trials was summarized in subsequent publications.[9] Worsening heart failure during a hospitalization for acute heart failure was analogous to reinfarction after an episode of acute coronary syndrome—a failure of the initial treatment strategy. This endpoint was a departure from traditional acute heart failure studies that focused on acute symptoms—primarily dyspnea—or postdischarge outcomes. Neither acute symptoms nor postdischarge outcomes capture the inpatient clinical course, a critical time for heart failure patients. The purpose of worsening heart failure as an endpoint is to represent the inpatient course in a way that can be measured in a clinical trial. Furthermore, in-hospital worsening heart failure is unique to episodes of acute heart failure. Recognizing the different physiology of acute and chronic heart failure underscores the need for different outcomes in clinical trials of these disease states.[10]

Despite the value of identifying worsening heart failure, there are also some challenges with using worsening heart failure as a clinical trial endpoint. Most notably, it may be difficult to ascertain whether escalation of care is due to true worsening of a patient's condition or due to initial undertreatment. This determination is particularly challenging for patients who are deemed

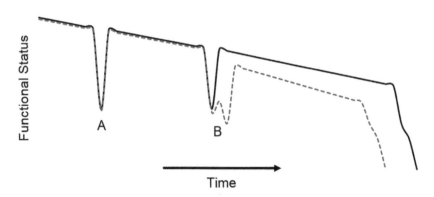

Fig. 1. Patient's clinical trajectory after an episode of in-hospital worsening heart failure (*dotted gray line*) compared with clinical trajectory without worsening heart failure (*solid black line*). The heart failure syndrome is characterized by acute changes in status typically requiring a hospitalization (*A*). In-hospital worsening heart failure (*B, dotted gray line*) represents a more complicated and costly hospitalization associated with worse long-term outcomes.

unresponsive to initial treatment and for patients classified as having worsening heart failure early in the hospital course.

INITIAL DESCRIPTIONS OF THE INCIDENCE OF WORSENING HEART FAILURE AND ASSOCIATED OUTCOMES

One of the first studies to examine the incidence of in-hospital worsening heart failure in patients admitted with acute heart failure was performed in a single-center, community hospital in Israel.[9] Patients were considered to have in-hospital early worsening heart failure if, from 6 hours after admission through day 7 of admission, they had "unresolved or recurrent symptoms and signs of heart failure that required an increase in or institution of intravenous heart failure-specific therapy, or institution of mechanical ventilatory or circulatory support."[9] They found that 29% of 337 patients experienced worsening heart failure, which was associated with increased mortality at 6 months (age-adjusted hazard ratio [HR], 3.3; 95% CI, 1.7–6.3).

The incidence of worsening heart failure and associations with outcomes was investigated retrospectively in early studies of tezosentan using a slightly different definition of worsening heart failure, which captured clinical events occurring both during hospital admission and in the early postdischarge period.[10] Specifically, worsening heart failure that occurred during the first 7 days of in-patient hospital admission was termed early worsening heart failure. In their study of 120 patients, 35% experienced early worsening heart failure during the first 7 days of hospitalization, and 7% required readmission within 30 days of discharge. Most in-hospital worsening heart failure events were treated with an increased dose of diuretics (82%). They found that patients with worsening heart failure were at higher risk of death at 6 months compared with patients without worsening heart failure (HR, 4.1; 95% CI, 1.3–13).

WORSENING HEART FAILURE AS A TRIAL ENDPOINT

Given the importance of identifying a meaningful endpoint for acute heart failure trials, and the proven association between in-hospital worsening heart failure and long-term clinical outcomes, worsening heart failure was incorporated into subsequent trials in acute heart failure, including VERITAS,[11,12] PROTECT,[13] ASCEND-HF,[14,15] DOSE,[16] REVIVE,[17] RELAX-AHF,[18,19] ROSE-AHF,[20] BLAST-AHF,[21] and TRUE-AHF[22] (Table 1). Each of these large clinical trials used different

criteria to define worsening heart failure, but all with the same general framework of a worsening clinical condition. Most trials also specified that the worsening clinical condition required an escalation of therapy to be considered worsening heart failure. The REVIVE trials, however, used only the clinical condition and did not require escalation of therapy.

The other differences between the trial definitions are mostly related to the setting and timing of worsening heart failure. VERITAS, RELAX-AHF, and BLAST defined worsening heart failure as occurring either during admission or early after discharge, whereas other trials defined worsening heart failure as occurring during index admission only. However, different trials focused on different timing of the occurrence of worsening heart failure. ASCEND-HF collected worsening heart failure events throughout the entire hospitalization, whereas DOSE and ROSE-AHF collected events from randomization through 72 hours, the REVIVE studies evaluated events that occurred after the first 24 hours and through day 5 of the hospitalization, and RELAX-AHF evaluated events that occurred through day 5 and also through day 14. Despite these differences, all of the trials included similar requirements for what constituted escalation of care. These treatments included initiation or increase of intravenous therapies for heart failure (including diuretics, vasodilators, and inotropes), implementation of mechanical circulatory support or ventilatory support, or the initiation of ultrafiltration, hemofiltration, or hemodialysis.

Recent guidelines from the European Medicines Agency regarding studies of medications for the treatment of acute heart failure state that for worsening heart failure to be used as a clinical trial endpoint, clear and objective criteria must be prespecified to reduce variability and inconsistency.[23] Although the Food and Drug Administration (FDA) has no such guidelines, they have raised similar issues for the worsening heart failure endpoint.[24]

ASSOCIATION OF WORSENING HEART FAILURE WITH CLINICAL OUTCOMES

From the clinical trial datasets detailed above, secondary analyses were performed to examine the association of worsening heart failure with clinical outcomes (Table 2). Worsening heart failure was found to be associated with worse in-hospital outcomes, including a longer length of stay, based on observations from the PROTECT pilot study and the VERITAS studies.[25,26] Data from the PROTECT trial showed the association between worsening heart failure and an increased risk of all-cause mortality at 14 days and 30 days.[27] The increased

Table 1
Worsening heart failure as a clinical trial endpoint

Trial	Year	Drug	WHF Endpoint	Definition/Time Course/Clinical Events	Treatment
Low-dose Tezosentan study[8]	2004	Tezosentan	Secondary endpoint: incidence and time to WHF or death ≤30 d after the start of treatment	Persistent signs or symptoms of HF in initial 24 h of treatment or recurrent signs of symptoms of HF, pulmonary edema, or cardiogenic shock after initial stabilization with 30 d of randomization	Initiation or increase of IV therapy Implementation of MCS or ventilator
VERITAS I and II[12]	2007	Tezosentan	Primary endpoint: death or WHF at 7 d (WHF during admission or after discharge)	Persistent signs or symptoms of HF with treatment or development of pulmonary edema, cardiogenic shock, or other evidence of WHF	IV treatment for HF (diuretic, vasodilator, or inotrope) Implementation of MCS, ventilator, or CPAP Use of ultrafiltration, hemofiltration, or hemodialysis.
PROTECT Pilot[25]	2008	Rolofylline	Primary endpoint: treatment success, treatment failure, or no change in condition	Worsening symptoms or signs of HF occurring >24 h after start of study drug to day 7 or discharge, whichever occurred first	—
PROTECT[13]	2010	Rolofylline	Primary endpoint: treatment success, treatment failure, or no change in condition	Death or readmission for HF through day 7 or worsening symptoms and signs of HF occurring >24 h after start of study drug requiring intervention by day 7 or discharge	—
ASCEND[15]	2011	Nesiritide	Secondary endpoint: composite of persistent or WHF and all-cause death	Typical clinical manifestations of worsening heart failure from randomization through hospital discharge	Addition or increase of IV pharmacologic agent Mechanical or surgical intervention Ultrafiltration, hemofiltration, or dialysis

Trial	Year	Drug	Endpoint		
REVIVE[17]	2013	Levosimendan	Primary endpoint: characterization of clinical course as improved, unchanged, or worse	Death through day 5 Persistent symptoms of HF from >24 after start of study drug through day 5	Rescue intervention specifically to relieve HF symptoms or Moderately or markedly worsened global assessment at 6 h, 24 h, or 5 d
Pre-RELAX[36]	2009	Serelaxin	Exploratory endpoint: in-hospital WHF from baseline to day 5	Physician-determined assessment on the basis of worsening symptoms or signs of HF	
RELAX-AHF[19]	2013	Serelaxin	Additional endpoint: time to WHF through day 5 and through day 14	Worsening signs or symptoms of HF	Institution or uptitration of IV therapy (furosemide, nitrates, other HF medications) Institution of MCS or ventilatory support
DOSE[16]	2011	Furosemide	Secondary endpoint: worsening or persistent heart failure	Need for rescue therapy within 72 h from randomization	Additional loop diuretic, addition of thiazide, IV vasoactive agent for HF Ultrafiltration MCS or respiratory support
ROSE-AHF[20]	2013	Dopamine or nesiritide	Secondary endpoint: worsening or persistent heart failure	Need for rescue therapy within 72 h from randomization	Additional IV vasoactive agent for HF Ultrafiltration MCS or respiratory support
BLAST-AHF[21] ClinicalTrials.gov NCT01966601	Ongoing	TRV027	Composite primary endpoint: time from randomization to WHF through day 5	Worsening signs or symptoms of HF during hospitalization, or rehospitalization for HF after discharge	Intensification of IV therapy including loop diuretics, nitrates, or other medications for HF MCS or ventilator support (including CPAP/BiPAP if used for HF)
TRUE-AHF[22] ClinicalTrials.gov NCT01661634	Ongoing	Ularitide	Coprimary endpoint: improvement in a clinical composite including WHF	Persistent or worsening HF requiring an intervention	Initiation or intensification of IV therapy MCS or ventilatory support, surgical intervention, ultrafiltration, hemofiltration, or dialysis

Abbreviations: BiPAP, biphasic positive airway pressure; CPAP, continuous positive airway pressure; HF, heart failure; IV, intravenous; MCS, mechanical circulatory support; WHF, worsening heart failure.

Table 2
Observational studies and secondary analyses of clinical trials assessing worsening heart failure

Trial	Year	Drug	WHF Definition	Outcome	Hazard ratio (95% CI)
PROTECT pilot[37]	2010	Tezosentan	Physician-determined WHF: worsening signs and symptoms of HF AND initiation or uptitration of IV treatment or MCS for HF	LOS 60 d CV/RF readmission and death	Mean (SD): WHF vs no WHF, 13.8 (6.8) vs 9.3 (5.9) 49.7% vs 19.5% in patients without WHF
PROTECT[27]	2011	Rolofylline	Worsening signs and symptoms of HF with resulting intensification of IV therapy for HF or MCS or ventilator support	14-d all-cause mortality 30-d all-cause mortality	6.84 (4.12, 11.35) 4.78 (3.10, 7.37)
PROTECT[30]	2015	Rolofylline	Worsening signs and symptoms of HF with resulting intensification of therapy: High-intensity therapy: initiation of inotropes, vasopressors and inodilators; MCS, ventilator support, and ultrafiltration Low intensity therapy: restarting/ increasing diuretics or initiating vasodilators without high intensity interventions	60-d CV/RF rehospitalization and death 60-d all-cause rehospitalization or death 180-d all-cause mortality 60-d CV/RF rehospitalization and death 60-d all-cause rehospitalization or death 180-d all-cause mortality	1.54 (1.22, 1.95), P<.001 1.55 (1.25, 1.93), P<.001 2.46 (1.87, 3.25), P<.001 High vs Low intensity 1.41 (0.88, 2.26), P = .15 1.32 (0.85, 2.05), P = .22 1.55 (0.93, 2.60), P = .096
Pre RELAX-AHF[28]	2010	Serelaxin	Worsening signs or symptoms of HF requiring the increase or reinstitution of IV therapy or MCS for HF	60-d HF/RF readmission or death 30-d all-cause mortality 60-d CV mortality 60-d all-cause mortality 180-d CV death	3.93 (1.72-8.98), P = .001 7.70 (1.72-34.41), P = .008 4.56 (1.02-20.20), P = .05 3.76 (1.23-11.50), P = .02 6.04 (1.75-20.87), P = .004
RELAX-AHF[38]	2013	Serelaxin	Worsening signs or symptoms of HF requiring reinstitution or intensification of IV therapy or MCS for HF	180-d all-cause mortality	1.90 (1.11-3.22), P = .016
PROTECT and RELAX-AHF[29]	2015	—	Physician assessment of worsening signs or symptoms of HF requiring intensification of IV therapy or MCS The treatment required was categorized as IV loop diuretic alone, IV inotrope (eg, dobutamine, norepinephrine, levosimendan, phenylephrine) or mechanical therapy (eg, mechanical ventilation, MCS, ultrafiltration), or other treatment (eg, IV nitrates, nesiritide, nonloop diuretic)	60-d HF/RF rehospitalization or CV death 180-d all-cause mortality	2.19 (1.80-2.67), P = .58 2.61 (2.20-3.10), P = .45

	Year			
VERITAS[26]	2014	Tezosentan	WHF could occur during the index admission or after discharge In-hospital: either (i) the development of pulmonary edema, cardiogenic shock, or other evidence of WHF or (ii) failure of the patient's HF condition to improve with treatment (treatment failure) Required at least 1 of the following: (i) initiation of new IV therapy, (ii) reinstitution of prior IV therapy, (iii) increase in current IV therapy for HF; (iv) implementation of MCS or ventilatory support, or (v) use of ultrafiltration, hemofiltration, or hemodialysis	LOS 30-d HF rehospitalization or death 90-d mortality	4.33 (3.54–5.13), P<.001 2.45 (1.75–3.40), P<.001 2.57 (1.81–3.65), P<.001
ADHERE[31]	2014	Registry	Any of the following criteria: initiated inotropic medications or an IV vasodilator >12 h after hospital presentation, were transferred to the ICU, or received advanced medical therapy after the first inpatient day	30-d mortality 1-y mortality 30-d all-cause readmission 1-y all-cause readmission 30-d HF readmission 1-y HF readmission 30-d Medicare payments 1-y Medicare payments	*Hazard ratio (99% CI)* 2.78 (2.55–3.04), P<.001 1.84 (1.75–1.93), P<.001 1.47 (1.35–1.59), P<.001 1.27 (1.21–1.34), P<.001 1.62 (1.43–1.84), P<.001 1.36 (1.26–1.47), P<.001 *Cost ratio (99% CI)* 1.70 (1.57–1.84), P<.001 1.43 (1.37–1.49), P<.001
ASCEND[7]	2015	Nesiritide	At least 1 sign, symptom, or radiologic evidence of new, persistent, or worsening acute HF requiring addition of a new IV therapy (inotrope or vasodilator) or mechanical support during index hospitalization targeted specifically at HF symptoms	30-d all-cause mortality or HF hospitalization 30-d all-cause mortality 180-d all-cause mortality	8.43 (6.70–10.60), P<.001 16.56 (12.58–21.79), P<.001 5.05 (4.23–6.03), P<.001

(continued on next page)

Table 2
(continued)

Trial	Year	Drug	WHF Definition	Outcome	Hazard ratio (95% CI)
ADHERE[6]	2015	Registry	Any of the following criteria: use of IV inotropes or vasodilators; mechanical support including ventilator, dialysis, IABP or LVAD; or an ICU stay during the index hospitalization	*Early WHF vs late WHF*	*Hazard ratio (99% CI)*
				30-d mortality	0.69 (0.57–0.83), *P*<.001
				1-y mortality	0.84 (0.75–0.94), *P*<.001
				30-d all-cause readmission	1.04 (0.91–1.20), *P* = .44
				1-y all-cause readmission	1.08 (1.01–1.16), *P* = .003
			Early WHF: occurred during day 1 of hospitalization	30-d HF readmission	0.95 (0.75–1.19), *P* = .54
				1-y HF readmission	0.99 (0.86–1.13), *P* = .81
			Late WHF: occurred after day 1 of hospitalization		Cost ratio (99% CI)
				30-d Medicare payments	1.09 (0.94–1.28), *P* = .14
				1-y Medicare payments	1.26 (1.16–1.37), *P*<.001

Abbreviations: CV, cardiovascular; HF, heart failure; IABP, intraaortic balloon pump; ICU, intensive care unit; IV, intravenous; LOS, length of stay; LVAD, left ventricular assist device; MCS, mechanical circulatory support; RF, renal failure; WHF, worsening heart failure.

risk of 30-day all-cause mortality was also observed in data from the Pre-RELAX trial.[28] In addition, worsening heart failure was associated with increased all-cause mortality at 60 days, 90 days, and 180 days, and cardiovascular mortality at 60 days and 180 days.[26,28–30] A recent analysis of ASCEND-HF confirmed increased risk of 30-day and 180-day mortality in patients with worsening heart failure compared with those without worsening heart failure.[7]

Extending the study of worsening heart failure out of the clinical trial space to provide real-world data from patients in the United States, worsening heart failure was recently examined in the Acute Decompensated Heart Failure National Registry (ADHERE).[31] This analysis confirmed the findings of increased all-cause mortality at 30 days, and also found an increased mortality at 1 year. In addition to the mortality findings, there was an increased risk of all-cause and heart failure readmissions at 30 days and 1 year. Using Medicare claims data, the investigators also examined the financial implications of worsening heart failure. Because of increased readmissions for patients who experience worsening heart failure, it is not surprising that after discharge from the index hospitalization, postdischarge Medicare payments were shown to be greater at 30 days and 1 year for patients with worsening heart failure compared with those without worsening heart failure.[31]

In an effort to further examine the condition of worsening heart failure, several analyses examined timing of worsening heart failure. Two studies, one using data from ASCEND-HF and one using data from PROTECT, stratified worsening heart failure by whether it occurred before day 4 of hospitalization or after that time.[7,30] There was no difference between timing of worsening heart failure and outcomes in these studies. A study using data from ADHERE categorized the timing of worsening heart failure differently. In this study, early in-hospital worsening heart failure was defined as occurring during hospital day 1, and late worsening heart failure occurring after inpatient day 1.[6] When defined by these time points, early worsening heart failure was associated with lower all-cause mortality but similar all-cause and heart failure rehospitalizations at 30 days and 1 year, compared with late in-hospital worsening heart failure.

Because worsening heart failure is defined by the need for escalation of therapy, 1 study delineated therapy as high intensity (initiation of inotropes, vasopressors, or inodilators; or initiation of mechanical support including circulatory support, ventilator support, or ultrafiltration) or low intensity (increasing diuretics or initiating vasodilators).[30] There was no difference between the groups in the risk of death or hospitalization at 60 days or death at 180 days.

TREATMENT OF WORSENING HEART FAILURE

Although many trials have included worsening heart failure as an endpoint, most treatments have not been shown to be associated with decreased worsening heart failure. Compared with placebo, tezosentan was not associated with decreased incidence of worsening heart failure (odds ratio [OR], 0.99; 95% CI, 0.92–1.21), nor was rollofylline (OR, 1.13; 95% CI, 0.90–1.42). Similarly, in ASCEND-HF, the composite endpoint of worsening heart failure or death during index hospitalization was similar for the nesiritide group (4.2%) and placebo group (4.8%).

Two drugs have shown an improvement in worsening heart failure in adequately powered clinical trials—levosimendan and serelaxin. In the REVIVE trials, the placebo groups had more patients classified as worsening clinical course compared with the levosimendan groups. However, this study noted serious adverse events associated with the drug. Levosimendan has not been approved by the FDA for an indication in the acute decompensated heart failure patient population; however, this drug is being studied currently for use in patients with reduced left ventricular ejection fraction undergoing cardiac surgery (ClinicalTrials.gov NCT02025621). In the RELAX-AHF trial, treatment with serelaxin decreased worsening heart failure through day 5 (HR, 0.3; 95% CI, 0.1–0.4) and day 14 (HR, 0.7; 95% CI, 0.51–0.96).[19] The worsening heart failure endpoint was exploratory and not prespecified. When serelaxin was evaluated by the FDA in 2014, the FDA report noted that the endpoint of worsening heart failure was not well-characterized in the RELAX-AHF trial.[24] A larger trial of serelaxin is ongoing, with worsening heart failure as a prespecified secondary endpoint (ClinicalTrials.gov NCT NCT01870778).

PREDICTION OF WORSENING HEART FAILURE

The frequent occurrence of worsening heart failure in patients hospitalized with acute heart failure, and the association of worsening heart failure with poor outcomes including rehospitalization and death, has motivated the development of worsening heart failure as an important outcome in the care of patients with acute heart failure and highlighted the importance of prevention of worsening heart failure in these patients. Using clinical trials and registries, several groups have developed prediction models for the development of worsening heart failure (**Table 3**). Predictors of death, heart failure rehospitalization, or worsening heart failure at 7 days in PROTECT and validated in VERITAS include blood urea nitrogen, albumin, and cholesterol, as well as heart rate, systolic blood pressure, and respiratory rate, with blood urea nitrogen being the strongest predictor. Using patients from both PROTECT and RELAX-AHF, predictors of death or worsening heart failure through day 5 included blood urea nitrogen, hematocrit, respiratory rate, and systolic blood pressure. A risk model developed in ADHERE and validated in ASCEND found several variables that were associated independently with the development of in-hospital worsening heart failure, including age, heart rate, systolic blood pressure, left ventricular ejection fraction, and the laboratory values of brain natriuretic peptide, troponin, sodium, blood urea nitrogen, and creatinine. The strongest predictors were troponin and creatinine. Taken together, it seems that renal dysfunction, cardiac injury, and markers of decompensation all predict worsening heart failure.

DEVELOPING THERAPEUTICS AND TREATMENT STRATEGIES THAT DECREASE WORSENING HEART FAILURE

From the first use of worsening heart failure as an endpoint in 2004, there is now a robust body of evidence linking worsening heart failure with poor future outcomes. This endpoint may offer significant advantage over other symptom-based and clinical endpoints.[32,33]

Acute heart failure is recognized currently as a heterogeneous disorder characterized by symptoms, typically dyspnea, and findings of congestion and/or poor perfusion that clearly represent a deviation from the typical journey of a patient

Table 3
Prediction models for worsening heart failure

Trial	Year	Outcome	Predictors	C-Statistic	External Validation (C-statistic)
PROTECT and RELAX-AHF[29]	2015	Death or WHF through day 5	Higher blood urea nitrogen Respiratory rate Hematocrit Systolic blood pressure	0.67	—
PROTECT[39]	2012	Death, heart failure rehospitalization, or WHF through day 7	Higher blood urea nitrogen Lower serum albumin Lower serum cholesterol Lower systolic blood pressure Higher heart rate Higher respiratory rate	0.67	VERITAS (0.67)
ADHERE[40]	2015	In-hospital WHF	Age Heart rate Systolic blood pressure Left ventricular ejection fraction Brain natriuretic peptide Troponin (positive or negative) Sodium Blood urea nitrogen Creatinine	0.74	ASCEND (0.63)

Abbreviation: WHF, worsening heart failure.

with chronic heart failure (see **Fig. 1**). The reasons for this remain incompletely understood, but therapeutics and treatment strategies are focused on restoring the clinical status of the patient, that is, relieving symptoms and improving congestion and perfusion. In-hospital worsening heart failure represents a failure of initial treatment strategies to achieve all of these clinical goals and is characterized by increased level of care, either medical therapy or mechanical circulatory support. Although clinical judgment is necessary for changing a level of care, this clearly documented and measurable event is representative of the many facets of the heart failure syndrome and incorporates resource utilization, an often overlooked aspect of clinical care.

The authors believe that worsening heart failure may have advantages over other acute heart failure endpoints, such as dyspnea. There are challenges with standardizing dyspnea measurements, and furthermore, although dyspnea is a patient-centered outcome, it only represents one aspect of the acute heart failure syndrome.[34] As worsening heart failure continues to be incorporated into clinical trials, we must recognize that a standardized definition is required to compare results across trials.[18,22] Given the continued emphasis on pragmatic clinical trials, this standardized definition of worsening heart failure should be simple and easily ascertained from electronic health records.[35]

SUMMARY

In-hospital worsening heart failure occurs when a patient hospitalized for treatment of acute heart failure experiences a worsening of their condition while in the hospital, requiring escalation of therapy. In-hospital worsening heart failure is associated with a worse prognosis, including worse in-hospital outcomes, increased short- and long-term postdischarge mortality, increased readmissions, and greater health care spending. Renal dysfunction, cardiac injury, and markers of decompensation are the strongest predictors of worsening heart failure. No drugs have been approved by the FDA for the prevention of worsening heart failure, but trials are ongoing. In acute heart failure trials, worsening heart failure has advantages over other endpoints commonly used in acute and chronic heart failure trials, such as dyspnea relief and mortality or rehospitalization, and should continue to be used as an endpoint in these trials. We must continue to test and evaluate treatment strategies and therapeutics for acute heart failure and we believe there is substantial evidence to support worsening heart failure as a trial endpoint in these clinical trials.

REFERENCES

1. Mozaffarian D, Benjamin EJ, Go AS, et al. Heart disease and stroke statistics-2015 update: a report from the American Heart Association. Circulation 2015;131(4):e29–322.
2. Ramirez A, Abelmann WH. Cardiac decompensation. N Engl J Med 1974;290(9):499–501.
3. Yancy CW, Jessup M, Bozkurt B, et al. 2013 ACCF/AHA guideline for the management of heart failure: a report of the American College of Cardiology Foundation/American Heart Association Task Force on practice guidelines. Circulation 2013;128(16):e240–327.
4. Solomon SD, Dobson J, Pocock S, et al. Influence of nonfatal hospitalization for heart failure on subsequent mortality in patients with chronic heart failure. Circulation 2007;116(13):1482–7.
5. Setoguchi S, Stevenson LW, Schneeweiss S. Repeated hospitalizations predict mortality in the community population with heart failure. Am Heart J 2007;154(2):260–6.
6. Cooper LB, Hammill BG, Sharma PP, et al. Differences in health care utilization and outcomes based on timing of in-hospital worsening heart failure. Circ Cardiovasc Qual Outcomes 2015;8(Suppl 2):A324.
7. Kelly JP, Mentz RJ, Hasselblad V, et al. Worsening heart failure during hospitalization for acute heart failure: insights from the Acute Study of Clinical Effectiveness of Nesiritide in Decompensated Heart Failure (ASCEND-HF). American Heart Journal, in press.
8. Cotter G, Kaluski E, Stangl K, et al. The hemodynamic and neurohormonal effects of low doses of tezosentan (an endothelin A/B receptor antagonist) in patients with acute heart failure. Eur J Heart Fail 2004;6(5):601–9.
9. Weatherley BD, Milo-Cotter O, Felker GM, et al. Early worsening heart failure in patients admitted with acute heart failure–a new outcome measure associated with long-term prognosis? Fundam Clin Pharmacol 2009;23(5):633–9.
10. Torre-Amione G, Milo-Cotter O, Kaluski E, et al. Early worsening heart failure in patients admitted for acute heart failure: time course, hemodynamic predictors, and outcome. J Card Fail 2009;15(8):639–44.
11. Teerlink JR, McMurray JJ, Bourge RC, et al. Tezosentan in patients with acute heart failure: design of the Value of Endothelin Receptor Inhibition with Tezosentan in Acute heart failure Study (VERITAS). Am Heart J 2005;150(1):46–53.
12. McMurray JJ, Teerlink JR, Cotter G, et al. Effects of tezosentan on symptoms and clinical outcomes in patients with acute heart failure: the VERITAS randomized controlled trials. JAMA 2007;298(17):2009–19.
13. Massie BM, O'Connor CM, Metra M, et al. Rolofylline, an adenosine A1-receptor antagonist, in acute heart failure. N Engl J Med 2010;363(15):1419–28.

14. Hernandez AF, O'Connor CM, Starling RC, et al. Rationale and design of the acute study of clinical effectiveness of nesiritide in decompensated heart failure trial (ASCEND-HF). Am Heart J 2009;157(2): 271–7.

15. O'Connor CM, Starling RC, Hernandez AF, et al. Effect of nesiritide in patients with acute decompensated heart failure. N Engl J Med 2011;365(1):32–43.

16. Felker GM, Lee KL, Bull DA, et al. Diuretic strategies in patients with acute decompensated heart failure. N Engl J Med 2011;364(9):797–805.

17. Packer M, Colucci W, Fisher L, et al. Effect of levosimendan on the short-term clinical course of patients with acutely decompensated heart failure. JACC Heart Fail 2013;1(2):103–11.

18. Ponikowski P, Metra M, Teerlink JR, et al. Design of the RELAXin in acute heart failure study. Am Heart J 2012;163(2):149–55.e1.

19. Teerlink JR, Cotter G, Davison BA, et al. Serelaxin, recombinant human relaxin-2, for treatment of acute heart failure (RELAX-AHF): a randomised, placebo-controlled trial. Lancet 2013;381(9860):29–39.

20. Chen HH, Anstrom KJ, Givertz MM, et al. Low-dose dopamine or low-dose nesiritide in acute heart failure with renal dysfunction: the ROSE acute heart failure randomized trial. JAMA 2013;310(23):2533–43.

21. Felker GM, Butler J, Collins SP, et al. Heart failure therapeutics on the basis of a biased ligand of the angiotensin-2 type 1 receptor. Rationale and design of the BLAST-AHF study (Biased Ligand of the Angiotensin Receptor Study in Acute Heart Failure). JACC Heart Fail 2015;3(3):193–201.

22. Anker SD, Ponikowski P, Mitrovic V, et al. Ularitide for the treatment of acute decompensated heart failure: from preclinical to clinical studies. Eur Heart J 2015; 36(12):715–23.

23. European Medicines Agency. Guideline on clinical investigation of medicinal products for the treatment of acute heart failure. London: 2015.

24. FDA. FDA Briefing Document, Cardiovascular and Renal Drugs Advisory Committee Meeting. March 27, 2014.

25. Cotter G, Dittrich HC, Davison Weatherley B, et al. The PROTECT Pilot Study: a Randomized, Placebo-Controlled, Dose-Finding Study of the Adenosine A1 Receptor Antagonist Rolofylline in Patients With Acute Heart Failure and Renal Impairment. J Card Fail 2008;14(8):631–40.

26. Cotter G, Metra M, Davison BA, et al. Worsening heart failure, a critical event during hospital admission for acute heart failure: results from the VERITAS study. Eur J Heart Fail 2014;16(12):1362–71.

27. Metra M, O'Connor CM, Davison BA, et al. Early dyspnoea relief in acute heart failure: prevalence, association with mortality, and effect of rolofylline in the PROTECT Study. Eur Heart J 2011;32(12): 1519–34.

28. Metra M, Teerlink JR, Felker GM, et al. Dyspnoea and worsening heart failure in patients with acute heart failure: results from the Pre-RELAX-AHF study. Eur J Heart Fail 2010;12(10):1130–9.

29. Davison BA, Metra M, Cotter G, et al. Worsening Heart Failure Following Admission for Acute Heart Failure: a Pooled Analysis of the PROTECT and RELAX-AHF Studies. JACC Heart Fail 2015;3(5):395–403.

30. Mentz RJ, Metra M, Cotter G, et al. Early vs. late worsening heart failure during acute heart failure hospitalization: insights from the PROTECT trial. Eur J Heart Fail 2015;17(7):697–706.

31. DeVore AD, Hammill BG, Sharma PP, et al. In-hospital worsening heart failure and associations with mortality, readmission, and healthcare utilization. J Am Heart Assoc 2014;3(4):e001088.

32. Allen LA, Hernandez AF, O'Connor CM, et al. End points for clinical trials in acute heart failure syndromes. J Am Coll Cardiol 2009;53(24):2248–58.

33. Felker GM, Pang PS, Adams KF, et al. Clinical trials of pharmacological therapies in acute heart failure syndromes: lessons learned and directions forward. Circ Heart Fail 2010;3(2):314–25.

34. Gheorghiade M, Adams KF, Cleland JG, et al. Phase III clinical trial end points in acute heart failure syndromes: a virtual roundtable with the Acute Heart Failure Syndromes International Working Group. Am Heart J 2009;157(6):957–70.

35. Butler J, Fonarow GC, O'Connor C, et al. Improving cardiovascular clinical trials conduct in the United States: recommendation from clinicians, researchers, sponsors, and regulators. Am Heart J 2015;169(3):305–14.

36. Teerlink JR, Metra M, Felker GM, et al. Relaxin for the treatment of patients with acute heart failure (Pre-RELAX-AHF): a multicentre, randomised, placebo-controlled, parallel-group, dose-finding phase IIb study. Lancet 2009;373(9673):1429–39.

37. Cotter G, Metra M, Weatherley BD, et al. Physician-determined worsening heart failure: a novel definition for early worsening heart failure in patients hospitalized for acute heart failure–association with signs and symptoms, hospitalization duration, and 60-day outcomes. Cardiology 2010;115(1):29–36.

38. Metra M, Cotter G, Davison BA, et al. Effect of serelaxin on cardiac, renal, and hepatic biomarkers in the Relaxin in Acute Heart Failure (RELAX-AHF) development program: correlation with outcomes. J Am Coll Cardiol 2013;61(2):196–206.

39. O'Connor CM, Mentz RJ, Cotter G, et al. The PROTECT in-hospital risk model: 7-day outcome in patients hospitalized with acute heart failure and renal dysfunction. Eur J Heart Fail 2012;14(6):605–12.

40. DeVore AD, Greiner MA, Sharma PP, et al. The ADHERE Risk Model for in-hospital worsening heart failure. Circ Cardiovasc Qual Outcomes 2015; 8(Suppl 2):A168.

End-of-life Heart Failure Care in the United States

 CrossMark

Jonathan Buggey, MD[a,*], Robert J. Mentz, MD[b], Anthony N. Galanos, MD[c]

KEYWORDS

- Heart failure • End of life • Palliative care • United States

KEY POINTS

- Patients with heart failure in the United States have high morbidity, mortality, and health care resource use at the end of life.
- Patients with heart failure have historically not routinely used palliative care and hospice services.
- The inclusion of palliative care and hospice services in patients with heart failure may improve symptoms, quality of life, and health care resource use.
- Mortality prediction models, standardized palliative care guidelines, and access to multidisciplinary palliative care services should be targeted for improvement.

INTRODUCTION

In the United States it is estimated that 5.7 million adults have heart failure (HF) and by 2030 more than 8 million will be affected.[1] The costs attributed to HF are $30.7 billion annually, with a large proportion of costs accrued at the end of life.[2] Much of these expenses can be attributed to high rates of hospitalizations,[2] and this trend is predicted to increase further over time, particularly among elderly Americans.[3] About 5% of these patients with HF have persistent severe symptoms despite maximal guideline-directed medical therapy (GDMT), and these patients are referred to as having advanced, end-stage, or stage D HF.[4] A minority of patients at stage D may be candidates for cardiac transplantation or recipients of destination-therapy ventricular assist devices (VADs). However, for most patients with advanced HF the focus of the goals of care shift from life-prolonging therapies to providing symptom management and improving quality of life, as captured in the concept of palliative care. Palliative care can be defined as a patient-centered, multidisciplinary approach to improving symptoms and quality of life, which does not necessarily exclude appropriate disease-modifying therapies.[5] Historically, palliative care has played a limited role at the end of life in US patients with HF,[6] but contemporary data suggest this trend may be changing.[7] The current American College of Cardiology Foundation/American Heart Association (ACCF/AHA) guidelines now suggest palliative care consultation as a class I recommendation for patients with advanced HF,[8] and since 2014 the Centers for Medicare and Medicaid Services (CMS) and the Joint Commission require a palliative care representative as part of the multidisciplinary team for VAD candidates.[9] This article reviews the available data for current management options, guideline recommendations, and current challenges for end-of-life care among the US HF population. It also highlights additional potential

Disclosures: The authors have nothing to disclose.
[a] Department of Medicine, Duke University Medical Center, Duke Medical Hospital, Medical Residency Office/Room 8254DN, 2301 Erwin Road, Durham, NC 27710, USA; [b] Division of Cardiology, Department of Medicine, Duke University Medical Center, Duke Clinical Research Institute, 2400 Pratt Street, Durham, NC 27710, USA; [c] Division of Palliative Care, Department of Medicine, Duke University Medical Center, PO Box 3003, DUMC, Durham, NC 27710, USA
* Corresponding author.
E-mail address: jonathan.buggey@duke.edu

Heart Failure Clin 11 (2015) 615–623
http://dx.doi.org/10.1016/j.hfc.2015.07.001
1551-7136/15/$ – see front matter © 2015 Elsevier Inc. All rights reserved.

heartfailure.theclinics.com

solutions to improve the incorporation of palliative care into HF management.

RESOURCE USE

There is a high rate of hospitalization near the end of life among patients with HF. An analysis of 47 patients with stage D HF not eligible for transplantation found a significant increase in costs and resource consumption the closer a patient was to death.[2] Using CMS data, the average cost of medical therapy in the final 2 years of life was $156,000, with patients spending about 1 out of every 4 days hospitalized in their final 6 months, during which they accrued more than half of their total costs.[2] The study results may have some limitations in the ability to generalize, because it was a small cohort of patients with end-stage HF. In addition, CMS data were collected retrospectively, and the applicability of a cost analysis more than 10 years old is uncertain.

However, more contemporary data have suggested that hospitalizations and outpatient visits for patients with HF in their last 12 months of life are declining, and use of palliative care services is increasing.[7] In Minnesota, 1369 patients with HF were prospectively enrolled from 2003 to 2011 and followed through 2012. The investigators reported an increase in hospitalizations at the end of life, and 82% of patients were hospitalized at least once in the final 12 months. However, from 2003 to 2012 there were fewer in-hospital deaths (33% vs 22%) and decreased rates of hospitalization (57% vs 46%) in the 12 months preceding death. Similarly, there were 32% fewer outpatient visits, but an increase in the use of hospice services (29% vs 42%) and palliative care consultations (11% vs 44%). Although the specific reasons for this trend among US patients with HF cannot be discerned from this single cohort study, it may be in part caused by more structured management strategies and guidelines, or it could represent a shifting cultural mindset surrounding end-of-life care. Overall, these data generate the hypothesis that the use of palliative and hospice care services may reduce hospitalizations and health care costs among US patients with HF.

PREDICTING DEATH

Although the 5-year mortality remains around 50%, survival after the initial diagnosis of HF has improved over time,[10] even among the elderly population.[11] Within the HF population, it is often difficult to identify patients who are nearing death, and patients are subject to an unpredictable disease trajectory. A national survey of general practitioners, geriatricians, and cardiologists found that only 16% stated that they could predict death at 6 months most of the time or always in patients with end-stage HF,[12] and patients tend to be overly optimistic when predicting their own survival compared with prediction models.[13] In order to correctly identify patients at the end of life and thus guide appropriate therapies, such as the initiation of palliative care, there has been an impetus to create accurate prediction models.

Hospitalized Setting

Using the acute decompensated heart failure (ADHERE) registry, which contains data on patients from 263 hospitals throughout the United States, investigators developed and validated a model that risk stratified patients and predicted in-hospital mortality using a patient's systolic blood pressure (SBP), blood urea nitrogen (BUN) level, and serum creatinine level.[14] Other tools have been created using different US registries,[15] and although these models are limited to the inpatient setting, they provide useful information to help guide hospital-based providers, patients, and families on decision making during an acute HF hospitalization.

After an HF hospitalization, short-term mortalities are high.[16] The organized program to initiate lifesaving treatment in hospitalized patients with heart failure (OPTIMIZE-HF) registry contains comprehensive data on patients with acute HF from 259 US hospitals.[17] An analysis of 4402 patients within the registry found that 60-day to 90-day mortality after hospitalization for acute HF was 8.6%, and 8 clinical variables were primary predictors of mortality, and these were incorporated into a risk score.[18] Another model created from a US-based trial to predict posthospitalization 60-day mortality included only 5 clinical variables: age, sodium levels, BUN levels, SBP, and presence of New York Heart Association (NYHA) class IV symptoms.[19] However, this scoring system and other models for predicting posthospitalization mortality[18,20,21] have had limited real-world impact and modest adoption into routine practice. In response, a contemporary model was derived from nationwide data on Medicare beneficiaries with HF and used variables routinely available in electronic health records (EHRs).[22] This model may be more amendable to EHR integration, leading to a more practical resource for predicting posthospitalization mortality in a US-based population.

Ambulatory Setting

In the ambulatory setting, one of the most validated and widely used models is the Seattle Heart Failure Model (SHFM).[23] It was originally developed in a cohort of 1125 patients with HF from the United States and Canada and was subsequently validated in 5 cohorts consisting of nearly 10,000 patients with HF. Although the model performed well in a US-based cohort of 4077 non–clinical trial patients,[24] a small European study found very poor correlation between the SHFM and observed mortalities of 138 community-based patients with HF.[25] Notably, more than 75% of the cohort had stage 3 or worse chronic kidney disease, and the SHFM does not account for kidney disease.

At present, a risk model with superior operating characteristics for predicting death has not yet been developed, and each of the contemporary models has limitations. For instance, almost all patients included in the models mentioned earlier had HF with reduced ejection fraction (HFrEF) and were usually trial-based patients, often yielding a younger patient population with fewer comorbidities. Similarly, most models are likely to underestimate mortality in patients with stage D HF, because this group is underrepresented in routine clinical trials. Thus application to the community-based HF population may be limited. Although models specific for patients with HF with preserved ejection fraction (HFpEF)[26] and advanced HF[20] have emerged, their utility has not yet been validated. Nevertheless, the use of such tools is a class IIa recommendation from the ACCF/AHA[8] and they can be used as one component of an overall risk prediction strategy. Although the accuracy may vary, these models may help stratify patients who have the highest risk of death. These high-risk patients should be considered for early targeting of appropriate palliative care services. An ongoing US-based randomized control trial of palliative care interventions among patients with HF is using the evaluation Study of congestive heart failure and pulmonary artery catheterization effectiveness (ESCAPE) risk score[20] to guide patient recruitment.[27]

MANAGEMENT OPTIONS

Management of patients with advanced HF can be broken down to life-prolonging and symptom control measures. Whether initiating or referring a patient for new therapies or discontinuing current therapies the first step should be a patient-centered conversation, involving shared decision making to further define the patient's values, goals, and preferences at the end of life.[28]

Prolonging Life

Although patients with HFpEF have similar 5-year mortalities to patients with HFrEF,[1] there remain a lack of therapies that have been shown to improve mortality and prevent hospitalizations.[8] Therefore, patients with HFrEF are discussed here. When considering therapy options, providers should ensure that patients without contraindications receive GDMT, including β-blockers, renin-angiotensin system inhibitors, and aldosterone antagonists,[8] as appropriate. As patients continue to progress despite GDMT, decisions to discontinue one or more these medications should be made on an individualized basis.[6] Providers must first have in-depth conversations with patients and their families regarding risks and benefits of continuing medications that could, for instance, worsen comorbidities such as depression, blood pressure lability, and renal failure.

Definitive treatment of end-stage HF requires cardiac transplantation or destination-therapy VAD. In the United States the number of adult candidates waiting for a heart transplant increased by 25% from 2004 to 2012, but donations have remained stable at around 3.5 per 1000 deaths, and thus wait times have continued to increase.[29] Mortalities are high while on the transplant wait list and nearly 10% of patients die within 1 year without transplantation.[30] Overall, only a small number of patients with end-stage HF are transplanted. For those who are, other issues must be considered before transplant work-up, including the need for lifelong immunosuppression, risk of graft failure or rejection, infection, malignancy, and other major complications.[31] However, other options, such as implantable resynchronization therapy and mechanical circulatory support devices, exist to improve symptoms and clinical outcomes.

VADs were originally designed as a bridge to cardiac transplantation but, with improvements in design and function, their use has evolved to include destination therapy in carefully selected patients with end-stage HFrEF.[8] In patients who are not candidates for transplantation, these devices are capable of improving mortality as well as patient-reported quality-of-life scores compared with optimal medical management alone.[32] The devices are associated with high rates of complications such as infection, bleeding, and device malfunctioning.[32,33] However, with the advent of continuous-flow VADs, patients have similar mortality and quality-of-life outcomes, but experience fewer complications, particularly device malfunctioning and sepsis, compared with pulsatile-flow VADs.[34] Given the complexity of decision making surrounding VAD placement, current ACCF/AHA guidelines recommend a multidisciplinary approach.[8] The early involvement of palliative care may improve a patient's postoperative care,[35] and in the United States the CMS and Joint Commission require VAD programs to involve a palliative care expert. Similar to other devices, issues often arise at the end of life regarding VAD deactivation. Other countries have had positive outcomes when preemptively addressing processes for device withdrawal as part of their VAD programs,[36] but this process is not routinely part of US-based guidelines.

The placement of an implantable cardioverter-defibrillator (ICD) has proven mortality benefits for primary and secondary prevention of deadly ventricular arrhythmias in the appropriate HFrEF population.[37] ICD therapy does not improve symptoms and has not been routinely shown to improve quality of life.[38] Patients who have received shocks report significantly worse quality-of-life scores and have increased mortality compared with those without a shock.[39,40] Patients need to be thoroughly educated on the role of the device before implantation. A US-based cohort found that patients with ICDs were not only undereducated regarding the devices but did not understand the option of deactivation as they approached the end of life.[41] This problem is further compounded by the fact that few physicians engaged in discussions regarding deactivation and often waited until the last few days of life.[42] Similarly, only 10% of US hospice facilities have policies in place to address device deactivation.[43] However, recent initiatives to improve physician-patient communication and foster appropriate ICD deactivation have been successful.[44] However, there remains a need for more widespread, standardized interventions to help guide interactions regarding the deactivation of an ICD as patients near the end of life.

Contrary to ICD therapy alone, cardiac resynchronization therapy (CRT) not only provides mortality benefit in select patients with HFrEF with widened QRS complexes but has been shown to improve symptoms and quality-of-life scores.[45,46] Recent data from 1820 patients (70% US based) with mild symptoms, an ejection fraction of less than or equal to 30%, and QRS greater than or equal to 130 milliseconds showed a significant reduction in HF-related events among patients with dual CRT/ICD function compared with ICD therapy alone.[47] This combined therapy, even in patients with less severe symptoms, may represent an ideal way to offer this class of patients with HF life-prolonging therapies that also provide symptom and quality-of-life improvement. However, many patients do not meet the specific requirements for implantation or may be nonresponders to therapy.[48] Questions remain regarding device management and deactivation as patients needing CRT near the end of life, but this has not yet been empirically evaluated.

Although numerous options exist to improve survival in patients with HF, each therapy also carries inherent risks. As patients near the end of life, there remains a need for providers to address discontinuation and deactivation of certain therapies and shift focus to symptom management. This shift is best accomplished with an early, patient-centered discussion, often led by a palliative care expert, which specifically addresses device deactivation near the end of life.

Symptom Management

A US-based study of patients with NYHA class III to IV HF found that lack of energy, dyspnea, feeling drowsy, and dry mouth were among the most commonly reported symptoms, and high symptom distress significantly correlated with worse quality of life.[49] In addition, the presence of depression is associated with a greater number of symptoms and overall symptom distress in patients with HF.[50] The main treatment of dyspnea is with diuretics, which do not have proven mortality benefits but can significantly improve symptoms.[8] Other agents that can improve dyspnea are vasodilators such as angiotensin-converting enzyme (ACE) inhibitors, nitrates, and hydralazine.[8] However, in patients with advanced HF, the utility of these drugs may be limited by persistent hypotension and renal failure. In patients who have refractory dyspnea despite these agents, low-dose opioids may improve symptoms,[51] and although often prescribed by palliative care specialists, their use has not been evaluated in a robust clinical trial and is not mentioned in US-based recommendations.[52]

The use of continuous intravenous inotropes as palliative symptom control in select patients with end-stage HF, despite optimal GDMT and device therapy, who are not eligible for either VAD or transplantation is a class IIb recommendation from the ACCF/AHA guidelines.[8] However, the agents' efficacies remain in question; for instance, a single study of 20 patients awaiting cardiac transplantation in Australia found that the therapy was safe, cost-effective, and reduced inpatient hospital duration,[53] but several US-based studies have found high mortalities with their use, thus questioning their safety.[54–56] However, other studies have found their use to be helpful in stabilizing patients near the end of life, and allowing them the opportunity to die outside of the hospital,[57] but potentially at greater overall financial burden because of the cost of the agents.[56]

Depression is common among US patients with HF and increases overall symptom burden.[50,58] Although depression is specifically addressed in the most recent ACCF/AHA guidelines, no specific treatment recommendations are given.[8] One of the only randomized controlled trials to assess pharmacologic treatment of depression in patients with HF enrolled 469 US-based patients in NYHA class II to IV with LVEF less than or equal to 45%.[59] Patients were randomized to sertraline or placebo for 12 weeks, and the study found no significant reduction in depressive scores or improvement in cardiovascular outcomes with sertraline. Post hoc analyses found that patients who achieved remission (regardless of the pharmacologic intervention) had fewer cardiovascular events and improved quality of life than those who did not.[60,61] Thus, although the optimal treatment options are not clear, it remains prudent for providers to address depressive symptoms as patients with HF approach the end of life, to potentially improve overall symptom burden and quality of life, and perhaps reduce adverse outcomes.

Improvement in quality of life is strongly correlated with improvement in symptom burden. It is recognized that patients with end-stage HF have as great a symptom burden as patients with cancer,[62] and, as they progress and life-prolonging therapies are deemed unavailable, it is crucial for providers to recognize and treat these symptoms, even if this requires discontinuation of other therapies.

PALLIATIVE CARE AND HOSPICE

Palliative care does not have to imply hospice care, although these two services are not necessarily mutually exclusive. In the United States, hospice care focuses on providing medical care, pain management, and emotional and spiritual care, without intent to cure, to patients who are deemed to have 6 months or less to live.[63] Despite the overwhelming symptom burden and decreased quality of life experienced by patients with end-stage HF, palliative and hospice care services have historically been underused.[7] Although use of these services is increasing in the HF population,[7] in 2013 there were 1.5 to 1.6 million US patients who received hospice care and only 13% had a primary diagnosis of heart disease.[64] Data suggest that patients with HF spend a median of 17 days in hospice, with 32% of patients receiving care for 1 week or less.[65] Proposed barriers to the use of these services include the unpredictable disease trajectory of HF, which makes predicting mortality in 6 months difficult; increasingly available advanced therapies; and inadequate training of providers to lead such transitions-of-care discussions.[66]

Overall, limited data exist on the impact of palliative care interventions in patients with HF. In a recently published trial, 232 patients with acute HF who were not actively dying or undergoing transplant or VAD evaluation were randomized to receive an inpatient palliative care consult or not, in addition to standard of care.[67] Patients who received palliative care consults had improved symptom burden and quality-of-life scores at 30 days after hospitalization, but had no differences in 30-day readmission or 6-month mortality. A pilot study of 20 patients with stage D HF who were referred for cardiac transplant found that palliative care consultation improved patient and family satisfaction.[68] Ongoing studies in the United States, such as the Palliative Care in Heart Failure (PAL-HF) Trial,[27] will provide important information regarding the efficacy and cost-effectiveness of palliative care services among the advanced HF population.

CHALLENGES AND SOLUTIONS

Numerous challenges exist to improving palliative and hospice care involvement in patients with end-stage HF (**Table 1**). First, it should be noted that access to palliative care and hospice services is variable across the nation.[69] Most hospice patients have a noncardiac diagnosis (often cancer), and patients with HF may have a unique set of symptoms, such as uremia, dyspnea, and depression, that require interventions that hospice programs are not always prepared to handle. For instance, many hospice programs do not accept continuous inotropes or multiple inotropes, but this decision varies between programs. Some palliative care programs also have less familiarity with using diuretics and opioids to manage symptoms of dyspnea or fatigue related to fluid retention. Management of sleep disordered breathing and the accumulation of fluid in both abdominal and pleural spaces may require additional device or drainage catheters for adequate symptom relief.

Potential solutions to improve the appropriate use of palliative care services include standardization of prognostic tools to allow early identification of patients likely to benefit from palliative care and hospice referral. Empirical data from trials such as PAL-HF will speak to the benefit of standardized models of care that include early palliative care involvement. There remains a need for patient-centered discussions of the optimal end-of-life management strategies, including device deactivation. Important data could be gathered using investigative resources such as The National Patient-Centered Clinical Research Network.

Table 1
Challenges and solutions facing palliative and hospice care in US patients with HF

Challenges	Solutions
Unpredictable disease trajectory	Improved and standardized mortality prediction models
Variable access	Increased number of hospice programs in rural areas familiar with HF Increased number of palliative care consult teams in hospitals with <300 beds
Unique symptom management	Improved education of hospice employees in management of HF-specific symptoms Broader use and financial support for the use of intravenous inotropes in hospice facilities
Lack of standardized recommendations surrounding end-of-life planning	Improved and more specific guidelines for providers explaining the need for earlier palliative care consultation Improved and more specific guidelines for teaching cardiologists how to talk to patients about palliative care and end-of-life issues Aggressive research examining outcomes when palliative care is involved in HF management
Limited reimbursements for end-of-life planning	Provide improved reimbursements for physicians who discuss both advanced HF therapies and advance directives Remove the stigma of discussing end-of-life issues with patients

Implementation of these tasks may be enhanced by improved public knowledge of common end-of-life issues, enhanced community engagement, and improved reimbursements for providers involved in end-of-life discussions.

SUMMARY

In the United States, HF is an increasingly common syndrome that is associated with high morbidity, mortality, and health care use. Overall costs and symptom burden increase as patients approach the end of life. Although numerous pharmacologic and nonpharmacologic therapies exist to prolong life, most US patients with HF may favor quality of life rather than quantity.[70] Although guidelines exist to encourage palliative care consultation for patients with advanced HF, the efficacy and cost-effectiveness of this strategy has not yet been proved, but available data suggest that it is feasible and effective. Although palliative and hospice care use are increasing, patients in the United States continue to underuse these services. The Institute of Medicine's 2015 study, *Dying in America*, suggests that Americans think that the medical system places too much emphasis on achieving cure and prolonging life and may cause unnecessary suffering.[71] Overall, there remains a need for reform in the way US providers approach and care for patients with HF at the end of life.

REFERENCES

1. Mozaffarian D, Benjamin EJ, Go AS, et al. Heart disease and stroke statistics-2015 update: a report from the American Heart Association. Circulation 2015;131(4):e29–322.
2. Russo MJ, Gelijns AC, Stevenson LW, et al. The cost of medical management in advanced heart failure during the final two years of life. J Card Fail 2008; 14(8):651–8.
3. Fang J, Mensah GA, Croft JB, et al. Heart failure-related hospitalization in the U.S., 1979 to 2004. J Am Coll Cardiol 2008;52(6):428–34.
4. Costanzo MR, Mills RM, Wynne J. Characteristics of "Stage D" heart failure: insights from the Acute Decompensated Heart Failure National Registry Longitudinal Module (ADHERE LM). Am Heart J 2008; 155(2):339–47.
5. Hauptman PJ, Havranek EP. Integrating palliative care into heart failure care. Arch Intern Med 2005; 165(4):374–8.
6. Goodlin SJ, Hauptman PJ, Arnold R, et al. Consensus statement: palliative and supportive care in advanced heart failure. J Card Fail 2004; 10(3):200–9.

7. Dunlay SM, Redfield MM, Jiang R, et al. Care in the last year of life for community patients with heart failure. Circ Heart Fail 2015;8(3):489–96.

8. Yancy CW, Jessup M, Bozkurt B, et al. 2013 ACCF/AHA guideline for the management of heart failure: a report of the American College of Cardiology Foundation/American Heart Association Task Force on Practice Guidelines. J Am Coll Cardiol 2013; 62(16):e147–239.

9. Modified: ventricular assist device destination therapy requirements. Jt Comm Perspect 2014;34(2): 6–7.

10. Roger VL, Weston SA, Redfield MM, et al. Trends in heart failure incidence and survival in a community-based population. JAMA 2004;292(3):344–50.

11. Barker WH, Mullooly JP, Getchell W. Changing incidence and survival for heart failure in a well-defined older population, 1970-1974 and 1990-1994. Circulation 2006;113(6):799–805.

12. Hauptman PJ, Swindle J, Hussain Z, et al. Physician attitudes toward end-stage heart failure: a national survey. Am J Med 2008;121(2):127–35.

13. Allen LA, Yager JE, Funk MJ, et al. Discordance between patient-predicted and model-predicted life expectancy among ambulatory patients with heart failure. JAMA 2008;299(21):2533–42.

14. Fonarow GC, Adams KF Jr, Abraham WT, et al. Risk stratification for in-hospital mortality in acutely decompensated heart failure: classification and regression tree analysis. JAMA 2005;293(5):572–80.

15. Abraham WT, Fonarow GC, Albert NM, et al. Predictors of in-hospital mortality in patients hospitalized for heart failure: insights from the Organized Program to Initiate Lifesaving Treatment in Hospitalized Patients with Heart Failure (OPTIMIZE-HF). J Am Coll Cardiol 2008;52(5):347–56.

16. Go AS, Mozaffarian D, Roger VL, et al. Heart disease and stroke statistics—2014 update: a report from the American Heart Association. Circulation 2014;129(3):e28–292.

17. Fonarow GC, Abraham WT, Albert NM, et al. Organized Program to Initiate Lifesaving Treatment in Hospitalized Patients with Heart Failure (OPTIMIZE-HF): rationale and design. Am Heart J 2004;148(1): 43–51.

18. O'Connor CM, Abraham WT, Albert NM, et al. Predictors of mortality after discharge in patients hospitalized with heart failure: an analysis from the Organized Program to Initiate Lifesaving Treatment in Hospitalized Patients with Heart Failure (OPTIMIZE-HF). Am Heart J 2008;156(4):662–73.

19. Felker GM, Leimberger JD, Califf RM, et al. Risk stratification after hospitalization for decompensated heart failure. J Card Fail 2004;10(6):460–6.

20. O'Connor CM, Hasselblad V, Mehta RH, et al. Triage after hospitalization with advanced heart failure: the ESCAPE (Evaluation Study of Congestive Heart Failure and Pulmonary Artery Catheterization Effectiveness) risk model and discharge score. J Am Coll Cardiol 2010;55(9):872–8.

21. Kociol RD, Horton JR, Fonarow GC, et al. Admission, discharge, or change in B-type natriuretic peptide and long-term outcomes: data from Organized Program to Initiate Lifesaving Treatment in Hospitalized Patients with Heart Failure (OPTIMIZE-HF) linked to Medicare claims. Circ Heart Fail 2011;4(5):628–36.

22. Eapen ZJ, Liang L, Fonarow GC, et al. Validated, electronic health record deployable prediction models for assessing patient risk of 30-day rehospitalization and mortality in older heart failure patients. JACC Heart Fail 2013;1(3):245–51.

23. Levy WC, Mozaffarian D, Linker DT, et al. The Seattle Heart Failure Model: prediction of survival in heart failure. Circulation 2006;113(11):1424–33.

24. May HT, Horne BD, Levy WC, et al. Validation of the Seattle Heart Failure Model in a community-based heart failure population and enhancement by adding B-type natriuretic peptide. Am J Cardiol 2007; 100(4):697–700.

25. Haga K, Murray S, Reid J, et al. Identifying community based chronic heart failure patients in the last year of life: a comparison of the Gold Standards Framework Prognostic Indicator Guide and the Seattle Heart Failure Model. Heart 2012;98(7):579–83.

26. Komajda M, Carson PE, Hetzel S, et al. Factors associated with outcome in heart failure with preserved ejection fraction: findings from the Irbesartan in Heart Failure with Preserved Ejection Fraction Study (I-PRESERVE). Circ Heart Fail 2011;4(1):27–35.

27. Mentz RJ, Tulsky JA, Granger BB, et al. The palliative care in heart failure trial: rationale and design. Am Heart J 2014;168(5):645–51.e1.

28. Allen LA, Stevenson LW, Grady KL, et al. Decision making in advanced heart failure: a scientific statement from the American Heart Association. Circulation 2012;125(15):1928–52.

29. Colvin-Adams M, Smithy JM, Heubner BM, et al. OPTN/SRTR 2012 Annual Data Report: heart. Am J Transplant 2014;14(Suppl 1):113–38.

30. Singh TP, Milliren CE, Almond CS, et al. Survival benefit from transplantation in patients listed for heart transplantation in the United States. J Am Coll Cardiol 2014;63(12):1169–78.

31. Lund LH, Edwards LB, Kucheryavaya AY, et al. The registry of the International Society for Heart and Lung Transplantation: thirty-first official adult heart transplant report–2014; focus theme: retransplantation. J Heart Lung Transplant 2014;33(10):996–1008.

32. Rose EA, Gelijns AC, Moskowitz AJ, et al. Long-term use of a left ventricular assist device for end-stage heart failure. N Engl J Med 2001;345(20):1435–43.

33. Holman WL, Park SJ, Long JW, et al. Infection in permanent circulatory support: experience from the

REMATCH trial. J Heart Lung Transplant 2004; 23(12):1359–65.

34. Slaughter MS, Rogers JG, Milano CA, et al. Advanced heart failure treated with continuous-flow left ventricular assist device. N Engl J Med 2009; 361(23):2241–51.

35. Swetz KM, Freeman MR, AbouEzzeddine OF, et al. Palliative medicine consultation for preparedness planning in patients receiving left ventricular assist devices as destination therapy. Mayo Clin Proc 2011;86(6):493–500.

36. MacIver J, Ross HJ. Withdrawal of ventricular assist device support. J Palliat Care 2005;21(3):151–6.

37. Moss AJ, Zareba W, Hall WJ, et al. Prophylactic implantation of a defibrillator in patients with myocardial infarction and reduced ejection fraction. N Engl J Med 2002;346(12):877–83.

38. Sears SF Jr, Conti JB. Quality of life and psychological functioning of ICD patients. Heart 2002;87(5): 488–93.

39. May CD, Smith PR, Murdock CJ, et al. The impact of the implantable cardioverter defibrillator on quality-of-life. Pacing Clin Electrophysiol 1995;18(7): 1411–8.

40. Poole JE, Johnson GW, Hellkamp AS, et al. Prognostic importance of defibrillator shocks in patients with heart failure. N Engl J Med 2008;359(10): 1009–17.

41. Goldstein NE, Mehta D, Siddiqui S, et al. "That's like an act of suicide" patients' attitudes toward deactivation of implantable defibrillators. J Gen Intern Med 2008;23(Suppl 1):7–12.

42. Goldstein NE, Lampert R, Bradley E, et al. Management of implantable cardioverter defibrillators in end-of-life care. Ann Intern Med 2004;141(11): 835–8.

43. Goldstein N, Carlson M, Livote E, et al. Brief communication: management of implantable cardioverter-defibrillators in hospice: a nationwide survey. Ann Intern Med 2010;152(5):296–9.

44. Kraynik SE, Casarett DJ, Corcoran AM. Implantable cardioverter defibrillator deactivation: a hospice quality improvement initiative. J Pain Symptom Manage 2014;48(3):471–7.

45. Cleland JG, Daubert JC, Erdmann E, et al. The effect of cardiac resynchronization on morbidity and mortality in heart failure. N Engl J Med 2005;352(15): 1539–49.

46. Bristow MR, Saxon LA, Boehmer J, et al. Cardiac-resynchronization therapy with or without an implantable defibrillator in advanced chronic heart failure. N Engl J Med 2004;350(21):2140–50.

47. Moss AJ, Hall WJ, Cannom DS, et al. Cardiac-resynchronization therapy for the prevention of heart-failure events. N Engl J Med 2009;361(14):1329–38.

48. Russo AM, Stainback RF, Bailey SR, et al. ACCF/HRS/AHA/ASE/HFSA/SCAI/SCCT/SCMR 2013 appropriate use criteria for implantable cardioverter-defibrillators and cardiac resynchronization therapy: a report of the American College of Cardiology Foundation Appropriate Use Criteria Task Force, Heart Rhythm Society, American Heart Association, American Society of Echocardiography, Heart Failure Society of America, Society for Cardiovascular Angiography and Interventions, Society of Cardiovascular Computed Tomography, and Society for Cardiovascular Magnetic Resonance. Heart Rhythm 2013;10(4):e11–58.

49. Blinderman CD, Homel P, Billings JA, et al. Symptom distress and quality of life in patients with advanced congestive heart failure. J Pain Symptom Manage 2008;35(6):594–603.

50. Bekelman DB, Havranek EP, Becker DM, et al. Symptoms, depression, and quality of life in patients with heart failure. J Card Fail 2007;13(8):643–8.

51. Jennings AL, Davies AN, Higgins JP, et al. A systematic review of the use of opioids in the management of dyspnoea. Thorax 2002;57(11):939–44.

52. Oxberry SG, Torgerson DJ, Bland JM, et al. Short-term opioids for breathlessness in stable chronic heart failure: a randomized controlled trial. Eur J Heart Fail 2011;13(9):1006–12.

53. Sindone AP, Keogh AM, Macdonald PS, et al. Continuous home ambulatory intravenous inotropic drug therapy in severe heart failure: safety and cost efficacy. Am Heart J 1997;134(5 Pt 1):889–900.

54. Gorodeski EZ, Chu EC, Reese JR, et al. Prognosis on chronic dobutamine or milrinone infusions for stage D heart failure. Circ Heart Fail 2009;2(4): 320–4.

55. O'Connor CM, Gattis WA, Uretsky BF, et al. Continuous intravenous dobutamine is associated with an increased risk of death in patients with advanced heart failure: insights from the Flolan International Randomized Survival Trial (FIRST). Am Heart J 1999;138(1 Pt 1):78–86.

56. Hauptman PJ, Mikolajczak P, George A, et al. Chronic inotropic therapy in end-stage heart failure. Am Heart J 2006;152(6):1096.e1–8.

57. Hershberger RE, Nauman D, Walker TL, et al. Care processes and clinical outcomes of continuous outpatient support with inotropes (COSI) in patients with refractory endstage heart failure. J Card Fail 2003;9(3):180–7.

58. Moser DK, Dracup K, Evangelista LS, et al. Comparison of prevalence of symptoms of depression, anxiety, and hostility in elderly patients with heart failure, myocardial infarction, and a coronary artery bypass graft. Heart Lung 2010;39(5):378–85.

59. O'Connor CM, Jiang W, Kuchibhatla M, et al. Safety and efficacy of sertraline for depression in patients with heart failure: results of the SADHART-CHF (Sertraline Against Depression and Heart Disease in Chronic Heart Failure) trial. J Am Coll Cardiol 2010; 56(9):692–9.

60. Jiang W, Krishnan R, Kuchibhatla M, et al. Characteristics of depression remission and its relation with cardiovascular outcome among patients with chronic heart failure (from the SADHART-CHF Study). Am J Cardiol 2011;107(4):545–51.

61. Xiong GL, Fiuzat M, Kuchibhatla M, et al. Health status and depression remission in patients with chronic heart failure: patient-reported outcomes from the SADHART-CHF trial. Circ Heart Fail 2012; 5(6):688–92.

62. O'Leary N, Murphy NF, O'Loughlin C, et al. A comparative study of the palliative care needs of heart failure and cancer patients. Eur J Heart Fail 2009;11(4):406–12.

63. Rubin R. Improving the quality of life at the end of life. JAMA 2015;313(21):2110–2.

64. National Hospice and Palliative Care Organization. NHPCO's facts and figures: hospice care in America. 2014. Available at: http://www.nhpco.org/sites/default/files/public/Statistics_Research/2014_Facts_Figures.pdf. Accessed June 13, 2015.

65. Bain KT, Maxwell TL, Strassels SA, et al. Hospice use among patients with heart failure. Am Heart J 2009;158(1):118–25.

66. Lemond L, Allen LA. Palliative care and hospice in advanced heart failure. Prog Cardiovasc Dis 2011; 54(2):168–78.

67. Sidebottom AC, Jorgenson A, Richards H, et al. Inpatient palliative care for patients with acute heart failure: outcomes from a randomized trial. J Palliat Med 2015;18(2):134–42.

68. Schwarz ER, Baraghoush A, Morrissey RP, et al. Pilot study of palliative care consultation in patients with advanced heart failure referred for cardiac transplantation. J Palliat Med 2012;15(1):12–5.

69. Lester PE, Stefanacci RG, Feuerman M. Prevalence and description of palliative care in US nursing homes: a descriptive study. Am J Hosp Palliat Care 2014. [Epub ahead of print].

70. Stanek EJ, Oates MB, McGhan WF, et al. Preferences for treatment outcomes in patients with heart failure: symptoms versus survival. J Card Fail 2000;6(3):225–32.

71. Institute of Medicine (IOM). Clinician-patient communication and advance care planning. Dying in America: improving quality and honoring individual preferences near the end of life. Washington, DC: The National Academies Press; 2015. p. 120.

Epidemiology of Heart Failure in Europe

Aldo Pietro Maggioni, MD, FESC

KEYWORDS

- Heart failure • Epidemiology • Prognosis • Guidelines

KEY POINTS

- Heart failure (HF) is a major public health problem. Patients admitted for acute heart failure (AHF) generally present with severe clinical characteristics and have a high in-hospital mortality rate as well as a prolonged length of stay, with, as a consequence, a strong socioeconomic impact.
- For this clinical condition, therapeutic developments have been scarce in the past decades. For this reason, current guidelines are not including recommendations based on solid evidences from randomized clinical trials. Prospective studies focused on different AHF phenotypes to identify new treatment strategies are necessary to positively influence the poor outcomes of these patients.
- In contrast to AHF, chronic HF was the object of several successful controlled studies conducted in the past 30 years, which encouraged the use of drugs and devices able to improve the outcomes of ambulatory patients. In this clinical setting, the efforts should be focused on the appropriate and widespread application of the treatments recommended by the current international guidelines in the real clinical practice.
- For both patients with AHF and chronic HF, observational research remains an important research tool to confirm the results of the controlled trials in the real world, to collect periodic reports, and to assess the quality-of-care indicators.

INTRODUCTION

During the past decades, the interest in observational research by medical societies, health authorities, and drug or device companies has been rising for several reasons, including monitoring the incorporation of guideline recommendations, the need for identifying unmet clinical needs, use of the observational data as platform for Continuous Medical Education, and health authorities' implementation of policies.

Several studies have been conducted in patients with HF, particularly in those with AHF, showing frequently conflicting results also in terms of relevant outcome measures such as in-hospital mortality[1-10]; this was mainly because of the different selection of patients and participating centers. Moreover, most studies had a transversal design with no or limited longitudinal observation and very infrequently enrolled patients with AHF and chronic HF in the same setting.

In Europe, nationwide observational studies have been performed by implementing a network of enrolling centers of different complexity balanced with respect to the hospital national networks with the inclusion of both patients with AHF and chronic HF in sizable samples, enrolled in the same centers and with a systematic 1-year follow-up data collection. This methodology allowed the investigation of clinical profiles, contemporary treatment, outcome rates, and their predictors in both AHF and chronic HF cohorts.

This article aims to describe the clinical profile and the short- and long-term outcomes of patients admitted to hospital for an AHF episode and of those with chronic HF.

Disclosure statement: the author has nothing to disclose.
ANMCO Research Center, Via La Marmora 34, Florence 50121, Italy
E-mail address: maggioni@anmco.it

Heart Failure Clin 11 (2015) 625–635
http://dx.doi.org/10.1016/j.hfc.2015.07.015
1551-7136/15/$ – see front matter © 2015 Elsevier Inc. All rights reserved.

The data are from 2 recent observational studies that provided reliable information on these topics: the Italian Network on Heart Failure (IN-HF) Outcome Registry[11] and the heart failure registry of the European Society of Cardiology (ESC) (European Society of Cardiology Heart Failure [ESC-HF] Registry).[12,13]

PATIENTS HOSPITALIZED FOR ACUTE HEART FAILURE

AHF is a complex, heterogeneous, clinical syndrome, often life threatening and requiring urgent therapy.[14,15]

Despite the relevant burden of this clinical condition, therapeutic developments have been scarce in the past couple of decades; as a consequence, current guidelines cannot include evidence-based recommendations based on solid evidences.[16,17]

For this reason, patients with HF remain at substantial risk for recurrent acute exacerbations and death.[2,5,18] Furthermore, local conditions leading to hospitalization of patients with HF, as well as their in-hospital care, may be hugely different in various countries and can change over time.[19]

Italian Network on Heart Failure Outcome Registry Findings

The registry included 5610 patients with HF: 1855 patients were admitted for AHF; 43.0% of patients were classified as having de novo HF and 57.0% as having worsening HF.[11,20]

According to the ESC guidelines used at the time of data collection,[21] the AHF profiles at entry were classified as acute pulmonary edema in 27.0%, cardiogenic shock in 2.3%, decompensated HF in 43.9%, right-sided HF in 8.8%, and HF in the context of acute coronary syndrome in 12.9% of patients; hypertension was interpreted as the cause of decompensation in 5.1% of the patients. This classification does not seem to be really useful to guide diagnostic and therapeutic procedures; consequently, the more recent ESC guidelines do not mention it anymore.[16]

Demographics, clinical history, and clinical data on admission of patients included in the IN-HF Outcome Registry are reported in **Table 1**. The mean age was 72 ± 12 years (range 21–98 years), and 40% were women. Ischemic etiology was significantly higher in the worsening HF group. Comorbidities such as chronic obstructive pulmonary disease, diabetes, and history of renal failure or atrial fibrillation (AF) were more frequent in worsening HF; in contrast, entry systolic blood

pressure (SBP), heart rate, and left ventricular ejection fraction (LVEF) were significantly higher in patients with de novo HF. An implantable cardioverter-defibrillator and/or cardiac resynchronization therapy was present in 13.3% of cases (21.1% in patients with worsening HF compared with 2.9% in those with de novo HF, P<.0001). The large majority of patients had signs of peripheral and/or pulmonary congestion.

The biohumoral data are reported in **Table 2**. Anemia was observed in 38.7% of the patients. Almost 55% showed an estimated glomerular filtration rate (eGFR; Modification of Diet in Renal Disease method) less than 60 mL/min/1.73 m^2 and 13.1% of the patients had severe renal dysfunction (eGFR <30 mL/min/1.73 m^2), mainly in the worsening HF group. When measured, the median values of N-terminal pro-brain natriuretic peptide (NT-proBNP) or brain natriuretic peptide (BNP) were elevated, and they were similar in the worsening and de novo HF groups. In the de novo group, the level of high-sensitivity C-reactive protein, as a possible index of inflammation, was higher than in patients with worsening HF. An electrocardiogram (ECG) was available for 1779 patients (95.9%), showing AF in one-third of the subjects (31.5%). The result of ECG was defined as normal in only 2.3% of the entire population. When considering echocardiographic parameters (see **Table 2**), the worsening HF group showed a larger proportion of patients with a severely reduced LVEF (<30%) and with severe mitral regurgitation.

In this registry, the median time spent in hospital was 10 days (interquartile range [IQR] 7–15); 51.9% of patients (46.5% and 59.1% of those with worsening and de novo HF, respectively, P<.0001) were admitted to the intensive coronary care unit (ICCU) for a median time of 4 days (IQR 3–7). Despite (or as a consequence of) a greater number of admissions to ICCU, patients with de novo HF spent less time in hospital [9 (IQR 6–14) vs 10 (IQR 7–16) days, P = .0001]. The all-cause in-hospital death rate was 6.4% (almost 90% cardiac), and it was not different in the worsening and de novo HF groups (6.0 vs 6.9, respectively, P = .41). As reported in **Fig. 1**, patients with cardiogenic shock had the highest mortality rate (23.8%), followed by those with acute coronary syndrome (13.0%), whereas patients with hypertensive HF had the lowest death rate (3.2%).

No significant differences in mortality were observed between the worsening and de novo HF groups. Patients admitted with HF and acute coronary syndrome are not mentioned in previous registries, but their risk of in-hospital death seems

Table 1
IN-HF Outcome Registry: clinical characteristics

	Total (n = 1855)	WHF (n = 1058)	DN-HF (n = 797)	P
Age (y), mean ± SD	72 ± 12	72 ± 11	72 ± 13	.14
Age ≥70 (y), %	64.4	65.8	62.6	.16
Females, %	39.8	37.2	43.2	.01
Ischemic etiology, %	42.3	45.3	38.4	.003
BMI (kg/m^2), mean ± SD	28 ± 5	28 ± 6	28 ± 5	.32
BMI ≥30 (kg/m^2), %	29.0	29.0	29.0	.78
Systolic BP (mm Hg), mean ± SD	134 ± 33	129 ± 30	141 ± 34	<.0001
Systolic BP < 110 (mm Hg), %	20.2	24.0	15.2	<.0001
Heart rate (bpm), median [IQR]	90 [73–110]	82 [70–100]	95 [80–116]	<.0001
Clinical History				
Treated hypertension, %	57.8	55.7	60.7	.03
Diabetes mellitus, %	40.4	43.0	36.9	.008
COPD, %	30.1	32.9	26.5	.003
Renal dysfunction, %	32.5	39.1	23.6	<.0001
History of atrial fibrillation, %	37.7	43.3	30.4	<.0001
Previous stroke, %	5.2	5.3	5.1	.89
Peripheral artery disease, %	19.8	21.8	17.1	.01
ICD in situ, %	9.5	14.8	2.4	<.0001
CRT-D in situ, %	3.8	6.2	0.5	<.0001
CRT-P in situ, %	1.6	2.3	0.6	.005
Signs/Symptoms at Presentation				
Pulmonary congestion, %	78.2	75.8	81.4	.004
Peripheral congestion, %	56.1	61.3	49.1	<.0001
Pulmonary and/or peripheral congestion, %	88.4	87.8	89.1	.40
Peripheral hypoperfusion, %	12.0	12.4	11.4	.53
Cold, %	10.8	11.1	10.4	.66
Somnolent, confused, sedated, %	11.5	9.6	14.1	.003

Abbreviations: BMI, body mass index; BP, blood pressure; COPD, chronic obstructive pulmonary disease; CRT-D, cardiac resynchronization therapy-defibrillator; CRT-P, cardiac resynchronization therapy-pacemaker; DN-HF, de novo heart failure; ICD, implantable cardioverter-defibrillator; IQR, interquartile range; SD, standard deviation; WHF, worsening heart failure.

Adapted from Tavazzi L, Senni M, Metra M, et al. Multicenter prospective observational study on acute and chronic heart failure: the one-year follow-up results of IN-HF Outcome Registry. Circ Heart Fail 2013;6:475; with permission.

severe (13.0%), confirming the need for a more intensive assessment and treatment.

European Society of Cardiology Heart Failure Pilot Survey

From October 2009 to May 2010, 5118 patients were included in the ESC-HF Pilot Survey.[12,19] **Table 3** shows the characteristics of in-hospital patients and compares it with those of ambulatory patients with chronic HF. In-hospital patients were generally older than ambulatory patients with chronic HF and were more often female. As expected, comorbidities were more frequent in patients admitted for AHF, whereas the rate of implanted devices was more common in patients with chronic HF. More than half of the patients with AHF had an ischemic etiology, confirmed by coronary angiography in 64% of the cases. In patients with chronic HF, an ischemic etiology accounted for just 40% of the cases, but angiographic confirmation was available for 85% of the cases.

At hospital entry, clinical signs of pulmonary congestion were detected in 62%, peripheral congestion was detected in 65%, and either

Table 2
IN-HF Outcome Registry: biohumoral data at hospital admission and echocardiographic findings

	Total (n = 1855)	WHF (n = 1058)	DN-HF (n = 797)	P
Hemoglobin (g/dL), mean ± SD	12.5 ± 2.1	12.3 ± 2.0	12.9 ± 2.1	<.0001
Hemoglobin <12 g/dL, %	38.7	43.6	32.2	<.0001
Creatinine (mg/dL), median [IQR]	1.2 [1.0–1.6]	1.3 [1.0–1.7]	1.1 [0.9–1.4]	<.0001
Creatinine >1.5 mg/dL, %	28.7	34.1	21.6	<.0001
eGFR <30 mL/min/1.73 m², %	13.1	15.3	10.2	.001
Glycemia >126 mg/dL, %	56.7	53.4	61.2	.001
Sodium <136 mEq/L, %	18.8	23.0	13.1	<.0001
SUN >50 mg/dL, %	57.5	64.6	48.4	<.0001
NT-proBNP (pg/mL), median [IQR] (n = 274 pts)	5168 [2518–11,583]	4496 [2461–9492]	5964 [2680–13,359]	.14
BNP (pg/mL), median [IQR] (n = 284 pts)	1112 [542–2225]	1200 [568–2314]	925 [540–2070]	.37
hsCRP (mg/L), median [IQR] (n = 389 patients)	7.0 [2.2–19.0]	6.0 [1.5–14.9]	9.0 [3.3–23.1]	.007
LVEF (%) (mean ± SD)	38 ± 14	37 ± 14	39 ± 14	.007
LVEF (%)				
<30%	29.7	33.4	25.1	.001
30%–50%	51.8	48.9	55.4	
>50%	18.5	17.7	19.5	
Severe mitral regurgitation (%)	22.9	24.5	20.9	.07

Abbreviations: BNP, brain natriuretic peptide; DN-HF, de novo heart failure; eGFR, estimated glomerular filtration rate; hsCRP, high-sensitivity C-reactive protein; NT-proBNP, N-terminal pro-brain natriuretic peptide; SD, standard deviation; SUN, serum urea nitrogen; WHF, worsening heart failure.
Adapted from Tavazzi L, Senni M, Metra M, et al. Multicenter prospective observational study on acute and chronic heart failure: the one-year follow-up results of IN-HF Outcome Registry. Circ Heart Fail 2013;6:475; with permission.

pulmonary or peripheral congestion was detected in 82% of the cases. Clinical signs of peripheral hypoperfusion were reported in 8.6% of the patients; 10.5% of admitted patients were described as somnolent or confused. At the ECG performed at hospital entry, AF was diagnosed in 35% of the cases and a large QRS (≥120 ms) was detected in 35.5% of the patients. An echocardiographic examination was performed in 75% of the patients. The median ejection fraction was 38% (IQR 27–52); 39.1% of the patients had a preserved ejection fraction, defined as greater than 40%. A moderate-to-severe mitral regurgitation was diagnosed in 43.4% of the patients.

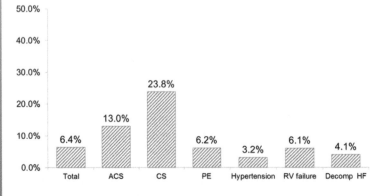

Fig. 1. IN-HF Outcome Registry: all-cause in-hospital mortality according to the AHF profile at entry. ACS, acute coronary syndrome; CS, cardiogenic shock; Decomp, decompensated; PE, pulmonary edema; RV, right ventricular. (*Adapted from* Tavazzi L, Senni M, Metra M, et al. Multicenter prospective observational study on acute and chronic heart failure: the one-year follow-up results of IN-HF Outcome Registry. Circ Heart Fail 2013;6:477; with permission.)

Table 3
ESC-HF Pilot Survey: comparison between AHF and chronic HF—baseline characteristics

	Pts with AHF (N. 1892)	Pts with CHF (N. 3226)
Age (y), mean $\pm$ SD	70 $\pm$ 13	67 $\pm$ 13
Females, %	37.3	29.7
Ischemic etiology, %	50.7	40.4
Documented by coronary angiography, %	64.0	84.9
SBP (mm Hg), mean $\pm$ SD	133 $\pm$ 29	125 $\pm$ 20
HR (bpm), mean $\pm$ SD	88 $\pm$ 24	72 $\pm$ 14
Treated hypertension, %	61.8	58.3
Diabetes mellitus, %	35.1	29.0
History of AF, %	43.7	38.6
Chronic kidney dysfunction, %	26.0	18.5
ICD, %	6.0	13.3
CRT-P, %	0.4	1.1
CRT-D, %	2.9	8.7

Abbreviations: CHF, chronic heart failure; CRT-D, cardiac resynchronization therapy-defibrillator; CRT-P, cardiac resynchronization therapy-pacemaker; HR, heart rate; ICD, implantable cardioverter-defibrillator; Pts, patients; SD, standard deviation.

Adapted from Maggioni AP, Dahlström U, Filippatos G, et al; on the behalf of the Heart Failure Association of the ESC (HFA). EURObservational Research Program: the Heart Failure Pilot Survey (ESC-HF Pilot). Eur J Heart Fail 2010;12:1078; with permission.

Anemia, defined as a hemoglobin level less than 12 g/dL, was detected in 31.4% of the patients; an eGFR less than 50 mL/min/1.73 m² and less than 30 mL/min/1.73 m² was reported, respectively, in 32.9% and 9.8% of the patients. NT-proBNP and BNP levels were measured at entry in 489 and 204 patients only, respectively. The median values were 4007 pg/mL (IQR 2043–9487) and 870 pg/mL (IQR 423–1950), respectively, documenting the severity of the clinical conditions at hospital admission.

According to the clinical profiles of the ESC guidelines,[21] decompensated HF (75% of the cases) was most frequent, while pulmonary edema and cardiogenic shock were reported in 13.3% and 2.3% of the patients, respectively.

Fig. 2 shows the overall rate of in-hospital mortality and that stratified by clinical profiles. Overall,

71 patients died during the hospital stay, the highest mortality rate being observed in patients with cardiogenic shock and the lowest in those with hypertensive HF. The cause of death was cardiovascular in 90.1% of the cases.

European Society of Cardiology Heart Failure Long-Term Registry

From May 2011 to April 2013, of the 12,785 patients screened for the study, 12,440 gave their informed consent and therefore became part of this analysis. Of these patients, 5039 (40.5%) were patients hospitalized for AHF, while 7401 (59.5%) were ambulatory patients with chronic HF.[13] **Table 4** reports the characteristics of the patients included in the registry. Patients included in the ESC-HF Long-Term Registry

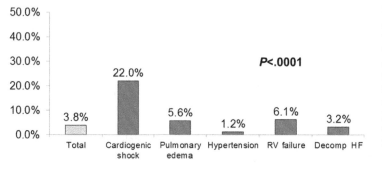

Fig. 2. ESC-HF Pilot Survey: total all-cause mortality stratified by the ESC clinical profiles. RV, right ventricular. (*Adapted from* Maggioni AP, Dahlström U, Filippatos G, et al; on the behalf of the Heart Failure Association of the ESC (HFA). EURObservational Research Program: the Heart Failure Pilot Survey (ESC-HF Pilot). Eur J Heart Fail 2010;12:1079; with permission.)

Table 4
ESC-HF Long-Term Registry: baseline characteristics

	HHF (N = 5039)	CHF (N = 7401)	P
Age (y), median [IQR]	71 [61–79]	66 [57–75]	<.0001
Age ≥75 y, %	39.5	26.0	<.0001
Females, %	37.3	28.8	<.0001
BMI (kg/m²), median [IQR]	28 [25–31]	28 [25–31]	.0002
SBP (mm Hg), median [IQR]	130 [110–150]	120 [110–136]	<.0001
SBP ≤110 mm Hg, %	27	31	<.0001
HR (bpm), median [IQR]	88 [73–104]	70 [62–80]	<.0001
HR ≥70 bpm, %	83.0	55.6	<.0001
EF (%), median [IQR] (available for 9722 pts)	38 [30–51]	35 [28–45]	<.0001
EF >45%, %	32.8	23.1	<.0001
NYHA III–IV, %	85.9	25.3	<.0001
Pulmonary or peripheral congestion, %	85.0	74.7	<.0001
Sound 3, %	32.5	5.8	<.0001
Peripheral hypoperfusion/cold, %	16.5	3.5	<.0001
Mitral regurgitation, %	44.4	26.2	<.0001
Aortic stenosis, %	9.4	3.9	<.0001
Prior hospitalization, %	29.8	40.9	<.0001
HF diagnosis >12 mo, %	54.5	63.9	<.0001
Ischemic etiology, %	54.0	43.0	<.0001
AF, %	44.0	37.6	<.0001
Diabetes mellitus, %	38.9	31.8	<.0001
PAD, %	14.2	12.3	.0021
Hypertension, %	64.5	58.2	<.0001
COPD, %	20.2	13.8	<.0001
Sleep apnea, %	3.0	5.2	<.0001
Prior stroke/TIA, %	13.0	9.4	<.0001
Renal dysfunction, %	26.4	18.2	<.0001
Hepatic dysfunction, %	8.4	3.4	<.0001
Depression, %	7.9	7.6	.553
PM, %	6.2	5.8	<.0001
CRT-P, %	0.6	2.3	—
CRT-D, %	3.1	11.0	—
ICD, %	4.8	15.9	—

Abbreviations: BMI, body mass index; CHF, chronic heart failure; COPD, chronic obstructive pulmonary disease; CRT-D, cardiac resynchronization therapy-defibrillator; CRT-P, cardiac resynchronization therapy-pacemaker; EF, ejection fraction; HHF, hospitalized heart failure; HR, heart rate; ICD, implantable cardioverter-defibrillator; IQR, interquartile range; NYHA, New York Heart Association; PAD, peripheral artery disease; PM, pacemaker; pts, patients; TIA, transient ischemic attack.

Adapted from Maggioni AP, Anker S, Dahlström U, et al. Are hospitalized or ambulatory patients with heart failure treated in accordance with European Society of Cardiology guidelines? Evidence from 12 440 patients of the ESC Heart Failure Long-Term Registry. Eur J Heart Fail 2013;15:1175; with permission.

present with baseline characteristics, clinical history, and comorbidities, which largely overlaps with the observations of other European or US registries.[1,3,12,22,23]

Patients hospitalized for AHF show a more severe clinical profile, as well as a higher rate of comorbidities, than patients with chronic HF, showing the substantial similarity of this population of patients with respect to previous reports.

To summarize the findings presented so far, **Table 5** reports some selected clinical characteristics of the IN-HF Outcome Registry and the

Table 5
Patients characteristics in previous AHF registries and in IN-HF Outcome Registry

	ADHERE[3] (N = 105,388)	EHFS II[8] (N = 3580)	Italian S[23] (N = 2807)	OPTIMIZE-HF[5] (N = 48,612)	ESC-HF Pilot[12] (N = 1892)	IN-HF Outcome[11] (N = 1855)
Age (y), mean ± SD	72.4 ± 14	69.9 ± 12	73 ± 11	73 ± 14	70 ± 13	72 ± 12
Females (%)	52	38.7	39.5	51.6	37.3	39.8
Ischemic etiology (%)	65	53.6	46	45.7	50.7	42.3
Medical History						
Hypertension (%)	73	62.5	65.6	70.9	61.8	57.8
Diabetes mellitus (%)	44	32.8	38.4	41.5	35.1	40.4
Renal insufficiency (%)	30	16.8	24.7	19.6	26	32.5
AF (%)	31	38.7	28.4	30.8	43.7	37.7
Baseline Medications						
ACEIs/ARBs (%)	53	63	72.5	51.3	60	59
Diuretics (%)	70	71	81	65.7	68	64
β-blockers (%)	48	43	32	53.1	62	41
Digoxin (%)	28	27	NA	23.4	21	16
De novo HF (%)	35	37.1	44	11.7	NA	43
Cardiogenic shock at entry (%)	NA	3.9	7.7	NA	2.3	2.3
Hypertensive AHF at entry (%)	NA	11.4	NA	NA	4.7	5.1
Physical and Laboratory Findings						
SBP (mm Hg) (mean ± SD)	144 ± 33	135 ± NA	141 ± 37	143 ± 33	133 ± 29	134 ± 33
HR (bpm) (mean ± SD)	NA	95 ± NA	97 ± 22	87 ± 21	88 ± 24	93 ± 26
Creatinine (mg/mL) (mean ± SD)	1.8 ± 1.6	NA	1.7 ± 1	1.8 ± 1.6	NA	1.5 ± 1.0
LVEF (%) (mean ± SD)	34.4 ± 16	38.0 ± 15	37 ± 13	39 ± 18	38 ± NA	38 ± 14
HFpEF (%) (LVEF cutoff)	46 (>40%)	34.3 (>45%)	34 (>40%)	51.2 (>40%)	36.1 (>40%)	35.0 (>40%)
IV Therapy and Intervention						
Diuretic (%)	NA	84.4	95.3	NA	84.6	99.0
Vasodilators (%)	21	38.7	51.3	14.3	18.5	29.9
Inotropes (%)	15	29.8	24.6	10.9	10.5	19.4
Outcome						
ICU admission (%)	18.7	50	69	NA	48	51.9
Length of stay (d)	4.3	9.0	9.0	5.7	NA	10
In-hospital mortality (%)	4.0	9.0	7.3	3.8	3.8	6.4

Abbreviations: ACEI, angiotensin-converting enzyme inhibitor; ADHERE, Acute Decompensated Heart Failure National Registry; ARB, angiotensin receptor blocker; EHFS, EuroHeart Failure Survey; HFpEF, heart failure preserved ejection fraction; HR, heart rate; ICU, intensive care unit; IV, intravenous; OPTIMIZE-HF, Organized Program To Initiate Lifesaving Treatment In Hospitalized Patients With Heart Failure; SD, standard deviation.

Adapted from Oliva F, Mortara A, Cacciatore G, et al. On the behalf of the IN-HF outcome investigators. Acute heart failure patient profiles, management and in-hospital outcome: results of the italian registry on heart failure outcome. Eur J Heart Fail 2012;14:1215.

ESC-HF Pilot Survey patients compared with subjects enrolled in other US and European registries.[3,5,8,11,12,23]

The in-hospital all-cause mortality rate of the IN-HF Outcome Registry was slightly lower than that reported in a previous Italian survey (6.4% vs 7.3%) but still higher than those of the ESC-HF Pilot Survey[12] and US registries (4%) reported in **Table 5**. However, considering the differences in length of stay and the rapid discharge home in US hospitals, some deaths may have occurred some days later. This fact is supported by the analysis of the 3-month mortality, which seems similar in the European and US registries (about 13%).

AMBULATORY PATIENTS WITH CHRONIC HEART FAILURE
Italian Network on Heart Failure Outcome Registry Findings

The all-cause mortality rate at 1 year of patients with chronic stable HF was 5.9%, relevantly reduced with respect to the mortality rates observed in the previous decades.[11] However, it was much higher, as expected, in patients in New York Heart Association (NYHA) class III–IV than in those in class I–II (14.5% vs 4.1%, $P<.0001$). The etiology did not seem to have a remarkable impact on outcome. The death rate was higher, but not

statistically significant, in patients with ischemic etiology (6.5%) than in those with a nonischemic etiology (5.4%) ($P = .17$). Of the 222 patients with chronic HF who died at 1 year, 65.3% died due to cardiovascular reasons and 16.2% due to noncardiovascular reasons and in 18.5% of cases, the cause of death remained unknown. Among the cardiovascular causes of death, HF was the most frequent cause (62.1%) followed by arrhythmic deaths (15.2%).

The 1-year admission rate was 22.7%; only one-third (8.8%) was due to HF and 13.9% was related to other cardiovascular (8.4%) or different causes. The proportion of HF hospitalizations was higher in patients with severe HF, whereas in patients with ischemic etiology, the prevalent cause of hospitalization was cardiovascular but not worsening HF. The rate of use of the pharmacologic treatments recommended by the current guidelines was high at the entry visit and did not change during the follow-up period (**Fig. 3**).

In contrast to the AHF domain, rich in observational studies but poor in successful randomized controlled trials, in the past decades, several large randomized controlled trials, mostly successful, have been conducted in patients with chronic HF, whose results are currently incorporated in the international guidelines,[16,17] while few systematic observational studies have been reported. The IN-HF Outcome study shows 2 encouraging findings.

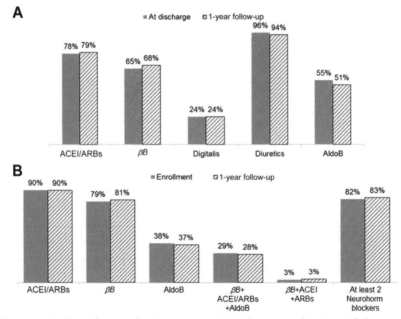

Fig. 3. IN-HF Outcome Registry: pharmacologic treatments at study entry and at 1-year follow-up. βB, β-blockers; ACE, angiotensin-converting enzyme inhibitor; AldoB, aldosterone blockers; ARB, angiotensin receptor blocker. (*Adapted from* Tavazzi L, Senni M, Metra M, et al. Multicenter prospective observational study on acute and chronic heart failure: the one-year follow-up results of IN-HF Outcome Registry. Circ Heart Fail 2013;6:478; with permission.)

First, the recommended pharmacologic treatments are incorporated in the clinical practice and maintained over time. Second, the evolutionary nature of chronic HF looks relatively controlled with an annual mortality rate lower than 6% (two-thirds for cardiovascular causes) in a population representative of the Western world with 17.9% NYHA III–IV patients and a median age of 71 years. Among the prognostic predictors of mortality, low SBP and low body weight are confirmed as alarming signals in patients with chronic HF, together with severe mitral regurgitation, anemia, renal dysfunction, and large QRS. High heart rate also emerges as an important marker of risk, with a 2% increase in probability of dying within 1 year per one incremental heart beat.

European Society of Cardiology Heart Failure Pilot and Long-Term registries

The rate of patients with chronic HF with moderate (NYHA class I–II) or severe HF (NYHA class III or IV) were 72% and 28%, respectively, of the total population of ambulatory patients.[12,13] An ejection fraction value was available in 2857 patients (89% of out-patients): the median ejection fraction was 36% (IQR 30–46), and a preserved ejection fraction was reported in 36.1% of the cases. A hemoglobin level lower than 12 g/dL was reported in 18.8% of cases, an eGFR lower than 60 mL/min/1.73 m^2 or lower

than 30 mL/min/1.73 m^2 was reported, respectively, in 40.7% and 5.1% of patients. NT-pro BNP or BNP levels were measured in a minority of cases (747 and 285 patients, respectively). Median values were 1387 (IQR 485–3381) and 390 pg/mL (IQR 133–870), respectively.

A blocker of the renin-angiotensin system, a β-blocker, and an aldosterone blocker were prescribed respectively in 89%, 87%, and 44% of the cases, respectively. The combination of a renin-angiotensin system blocker, a β-blocker, and an aldosterone blocker was prescribed in 35% of patients, while the combination of a β-blocker, an angiotensin-converting enzyme (ACE) inhibitor, and an angiotensin receptor blocker was prescribed in just 3% of the patients. Ramipril and enalapril were the most prescribed ACE inhibitors; the target dose of these drugs was used in 38.2% and 46.2% of the cases, respectively. With respect to angiotensin receptor blockers, the target dose of candesartan, losartan, and valsartan was reached in 28.0, 19.7%, and 16.7% of cases, respectively. The target dosage of carvedilol, bisoprolol, and metoprolol was reached in 37.3, 20.7%, and 21.4% of patients, while target dosages of spironolactone, canrenone, or eplerenone were prescribed in 22.2, 61.3%, and 32.7% of patients, respectively.

The all-cause mortality rate at 1 year of patients with chronic stable HF was 7.2% (**Fig. 4**). Patients in NYHA class III–IV showed a much higher mortality

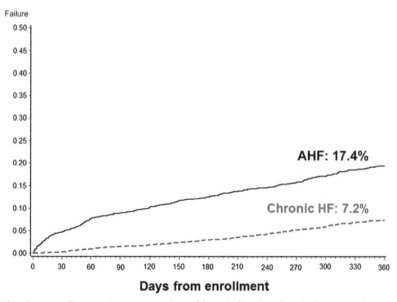

Days from enrollment

Fig. 4. ESC-HF Pilot Survey: all-cause 1-year mortality of hospitalized and ambulatory patients with chronic HF. (*Adapted from* Maggioni AP, Dahlström U, Filippatos G, et al; on the behalf of the Heart Failure Association of the ESC (HFA). EURObservational Research Program: the Heart Failure Pilot Survey (ESC-HF Pilot). Eur J Heart Fail 2013;15:812; with permission.)

than those in class I–II (13.5% vs 4.8%, $P<.0001$). Of the 233 patients with chronic HF who died at 1 year, 54.5% died due to cardiovascular reasons and 16.3% due to noncardiovascular reasons and in 29.2% of cases, the cause of death remained unknown. Among the cardiac causes of death, sudden death occurred in 40.2% of the cases.

The 1-year admission rate was 31.9%, 24.0% for cardiovascular reasons and 11.4% for non-cardiovascular reasons. Of all admissions, 41.7% were due to HF.

SUMMARY

While death rate of patients with chronic HF seems to slowly improve over time, outcome rates of patients admitted for AHF are still unacceptably high. AHF remains a major public health problem, and the data reported here confirms the strong socio-economic impact of this clinical condition.

In the past 3 decades, there has been a small improvement in this field, and probably the most important issue to consider is that AHF is not a single entity with a unique cause but a spectrum of complex multisystem pathologies. The treatment is still largely empirical and has been practically unchanged for many years; the recommendations of guidelines are largely based on observational data or expert consensus. Undoubtedly, it is time to dedicate more resources to this field; prospective studies focused on careful description of AHF phenotypes, with measurements of levels of multiple markers during and after hospitalization, to improve understanding and identify new treatment strategies are needed.

With respect to chronic HF, the main goal of the various stakeholders should be obtaining the largest application in clinical practice of the treatments shown to be able to improve patients' outcomes. In this sense, a clear gap still exists between the recommendation of current guidelines and what actually happens in the real-world clinical practice.

Furthermore, no effective treatment still exists for patients with HF and preserved ejection fraction, who account for at least one-third of the whole population with chronic HF. Controlled studies in these patients are definitely needed.

Finally, the role of observational research remains an important tool to confirm the results of the trials in the real world, to collect periodic reports, and to assess quality-of-care indicators.

REFERENCES

1. O'Connor CM, Stough WG, Gallup DS, et al. Demographics, clinical characteristics, and outcomes of patients hospitalized for decompensated heart failure: observations from the IMPACT-HF registry. J Card Fail 2005;11:200–5.
2. Rudiger A, Harjola VP, Muller A, et al. Acute heart failure: clinical presentation, one-year mortality and prognostic factors. Eur J Heart Fail 2005;7: 662–70.
3. Adams KF, Fonarow GC, Emerman CL, et al, ADHERE Scientific Advisory Committee Investigators. Characteristics and outcomes of patients hospitalized for heart failure in the United States: rationale, design and preliminary observations from the first 100.000 cases in the Acute Decompensated Heart Failure National Registry (ADHERE). Am Heart J 2005;149:209–16.
4. Zannad F, Cohen-Solal A, Desnos M, et al, the EFICA Investigators. Clinical and etiological features, management and outcomes of acute heart failure: the EFICA cohort study (Suppl. Abstract). Eur Heart J 2002;4:579. P2978.
5. Abraham WT, Fonarow GC, Albert NM, et al, the OPTIMIZE-HF Investigators and Coordinators. Predictors of in-hospital mortality in patients hospitalized for heart failure: insights from the Organized Program to Initiate Lifesaving Treatment in Hospitalized Patients with Heart Failure (OPTIMIZE-HF). J Am Coll Cardiol 2008;52:347–56.
6. Cleland JG, Swedberg K, Follath F, et al. The Euro-Heart Failure Survey programme – a survey on the quality of care among patients with heart failure in Europe. Part 1: patient characteristics and diagnosis. Eur Heart J 2003;24:442–63.
7. Komajda M, Follath F, Swedberg K, et al. The Euro-Heart Failure Survey programme – a survey on the quality of care among patients with heart failure in Europe. Part 2: treatment. Eur Heart J 2003;24: 464–74.
8. Nieminem MS, Brutsaert D, Dickstein K, et al. Euro-Heart Failure Survey II (EHFS II): a survey on hospitalized acute heart failure patients: descriptions of population. Eur Heart J 2006;27:2725–36.
9. Siirila-Waris K, Lassus J, Melin J, et al, FINN-AKVA Study Group. Characteristics, outcomes, and predictors of 1-year mortality in patients hospitalized for acute heart failure. JAMA 2006;296:2217–26.
10. Harjola VP, Follath F, Nieminem MS, et al. Characteristics, outcome, and predictors of mortality at 3 months and 1 year in patients hospitalized for acute heart failure. Eur J Heart Fail 2010;12:239–48.
11. Tavazzi L, Senni M, Metra M, et al. Multicenter prospective observational study on acute and chronic heart failure: the one-year follow-up results of IN-HF Outcome Registry. Circ Heart Fail 2013;6: 473–81.
12. Maggioni AP, Dahlström U, Filippatos G, et al, on the behalf of the Heart Failure Association of the ESC (HFA). EUR*Observational* Research Program: The

Heart Failure Pilot Survey (ESC-HF Pilot). Eur J Heart Fail 2010;12:1076–84.

13. Maggioni AP, Anker S, Dahlström U, et al. Are hospitalized or ambulatory patients with heart failure treated in accordance with European Society of Cardiology guidelines? Evidence from 12,440 patients of the ESC Heart Failure Long-Term Registry. Eur J Heart Fail 2013;15:1173–84.

14. Rosamond W, Flegal K, Friday G, et al, American Heart Association Statistics Committee and Stroke Statistics Subcommittee. Heart disease and stroke statistics—2007 update: a report from the American Heart Association Statistics Committee and Stroke Statistics Subcommittee. Circulation 2007; 115:e69–171.

15. Gheorghiade M, Zannad F, Sopko G, et al, International Working Group on Acute Heart Failure Syndromes. Acute heart failure syndromes: current state and framework for future research. Circulation 2005;112:3958–68.

16. McMurray JJ, Adamopoulos S, Anker SD, et al. ESC Guidelines for the diagnosis and treatment of acute and chronic heart failure 2012: the Task Force for the Diagnosis and Treatment of Acute and Chronic Heart Failure 2012 of the European Society of Cardiology. Developed in collaboration with the Heart Failure Association (HFA) of the ESC. Eur Heart J 2012;33:1787–847.

17. Bonow RO, Ganiats TG, Beam CT, et al. ACCF/AHA/AMAPCPI 2011 performance measures for adults with heart failure: a report of the American College of Cardiology Foundation/American Heart Association Task Force on Performance Measures and the American Medical Association–Physician Consortium for Performance Improvement. Circulation 2012;125:2382–401.

18. Fonarow GC, Yancy CW, Heywood JT, ADHERE Scientific Advisory Committee, Study Group, and Investigators. Adherence to heart failure quality of care indicators in US hospitals. Arch Intern Med 2005;165:1469–77.

19. Maggioni AP, Dahlström U, Filippatos G, et al, behalf of the Heart Failure Association of the European Society of Cardiology (HFA). EURObservational Research Programme: regional differences and 1-year follow-up results of the Heart Failure Pilot Survey (ESC-HF Pilot). Eur J Heart Fail 2013;15:808–17.

20. Oliva F, Mortara A, Cacciatore G, et al, on the behalf of the IN-HF Outcome Investigators. Acute heart failure patient profiles, management and in-hospital outcome: results of the Italian Registry on Heart Failure Outcome. Eur J Heart Fail 2012;14:1208–17.

21. Dickstein K, Cohen-Solal A, Filippatos G, et al, ESC Committee for Practice Guidelines (CPG). ESC Guidelines for the diagnosis and treatment of acute and chronic heart failure 2008: the Task Force for the diagnosis and treatment of acute and chronic heart failure 2008 of the European Society of Cardiology. Developed in collaboration with the Heart Failure Association of the ESC (HFA) and endorsed by the European Society of Intensive Care Medicine (ESICM). Eur J Heart Fail 2008;10:933–89.

22. Mosterd A, Hoes AW. Clinical epidemiology of heart failure. Heart 2007;93:1137–46.

23. Tavazzi L, Maggioni AP, Lucci D, et al, on behalf of the Italian survey on Acute Heart Failure. Nationwide survey on acute heart failure in cardiology ward services in Italy. Eur Heart J 2006;27:1207–15.

Acute Heart Failure Syndromes in the Elderly
The European Perspective

Spyridon Katsanos, MD[1], Vasiliki Bistola, MD[1], John T. Parissis, MD*

KEYWORDS

- Acute heart failure • Elderly • European registries • Comorbidities • Prognosis

KEY POINTS

- Older patients have more comorbidities, arterial hypertension, atrial fibrillation, and heart failure with preserved ejection fraction (HFpEF).
- Older patients have increased in-hospital, short- and long-term mortality.
- Severe initial presentation and age itself worsens short-term outcomes; older age, renal dysfunction, and frailty are negative predictors in the long-term.
- The clinical profiles and management of elderly are similar in Europe and the United States, except for the length of hospital stay (LOS), which is shorter in the United States; there is common underuse of echocardiography in the elderly.
- There is underprescription of neurohormonal antagonists in elderly in Europe and the United States, but with improving trends.

INTRODUCTION

Although survival rates of patients with heart failure (HF) have improved in the recent decades, the prevalence of HF syndrome is paradoxically increasing.[1] This increase has been attributed to a combination of an aging population and the dissemination of effective therapies for HF. The elderly population is preferentially affected by HF with preserved ejection fraction (HFpEF), an entity with poor outcomes compared with HF with reduced ejection fraction (HFrEF) but with different phenotypic myocardial alterations and possibly different underlying pathophysiologic mechanisms.[2,3] In the real setting of acute HF (AHF), elderly patients—usually defined by a cutoff age of 70 to 80 years—constitute a considerable fraction of affected individuals: in large AHF registries, the mean age of patients with acute pulmonary edema or decompensated chronic HF was approximately 75 years, whereas the rates of octogenarians (≥80 years) ranges between 21% and 38% of the total population (**Table 1**).[4–16] Prospective registries and randomized clinical trials have reported notable differences between elderly and younger patients with AHF, most importantly regarding demographic data, clinical profiles, comorbid diseases, outcomes, and associated prognostic factors.[5–16] Age-related disparities also occur in the management of elderly AHF, as suggested by underuse of diagnostic modalities, guideline-recommended HF drugs, and other therapeutic interventions in the elderly.[17] In this review, the authors summarize current evidence from published registries and posthoc analyses of randomized trials addressing the specific features of AHF in the elderly and attempt to identify country-specific variations in aspects of clinical presentation and management by comparing results from the studies conducted in Europe and the United States.

Heart Failure Unit, Attikon University Hospital, 1 Rimini Str., 12462 Chaidari, Athens, Greece
[1] These authors contributed equally to this article.
* Corresponding author. Navarinou 13, 15122, Maroussi, Athens, Greece.
E-mail address: jparissis@yahoo.com

Heart Failure Clin 11 (2015) 637–645
http://dx.doi.org/10.1016/j.hfc.2015.07.010
1551-7136/15/$ – see front matter © 2015 Elsevier Inc. All rights reserved.

Table 1
Summary of studies comparing elderly versus younger patients with AHF

	Pulignano et al,[9] Prospective Registry (Italy)	Mahjoub et al,[16] Prospective Registry (France)	Fonarow et al,[15] Prospective Registry (OPTIMIZE-HF) (United States)	Metra et al,[11] Randomized Trial (VERITAS)	Komajda M et al,[12] Prospective Registry (EHFS II) (Europe)	Herrero-Puente et al,[8] Prospective Registry (Spain)	Metra et al,[14] Randomized Trial (PROTECT)
Date	1995–1998	2000	2003–2004	2003–2005	2004–2005	2007	2007–2009
Patients (N)	3327	799	48,612	1347	3577	942	2033
Age cutoff (y); %	<70; 69 ≥70; 31	<80; 61.9 ≥80; 38.1	<75; 47.2 ≥75; 52.8	<72; 47.3 ≥72; 52.7	<80; 79 ≥80; 21	<80; 48.3 ≥80; 51.7	<80; 79.1 ≥80; 20.9
Male	78.7 64.7[a]	59.9 37.4[a]	56.2 41.1[a]	69.4 49.9[a]	66 44[a]	54.7 39.6[a]	21.5 11.2[a]
BMI or weight	NA NA	NA NA	90.2 kg 71.2 kg[a]	30.7 27.1[a]	26.9 26[a]	NA NA	NA NA[b]
CAD	37.8 50.4[a]	34.4 43.3[a]	43.7 47.5[a]	NA NA	54 51	38.8 29.5[a]	6.7 3.4[a]
AF	19.2 30.7[a]	30.4 37.4[a]	21.7 39[a]	22.9 30.1[a]	36 48[a]	39.4 48.8[a]	12.9 14.5[a]
Hypertension	8.5 9.1	31 40.7[a]	71.9 70.1[a]	75.5 82.7[a]	61 67[a]	77 81.8[a]	NA NA[b]
Diabetes	NA NA	30 15.7[a]	27.3 22.8[a]	52.1 43.7[a]	34 29	50.1 34.5	12.1 8[a]
COPD	NA NA	20.9 17.4	27.4 27.8	18.4 20.2	19 22[a]	18.7 23.7[a]	5.4 3.4[a]
Available echo	67 61[a]	88.9 68.5[a]	88.4 84.8[a]	100% 100%	92 81[a]	39.6 29.9[a]	NA NA
HFpEF	22.6 32.6[a]	53 61.2[a]	40.8 55.3[a]	0% 0%	28 39[a]	32.3 48.3[a]	NA NA[b]
LVEF cutoff	≥40%	≥50%	≥40	≥40% or WMI<1.2	≥45%	Not mentioned	≥40
ACE inhibitors/ARBs	84.7 74.9[a]	68 42[a]	84.3 78.8[a]	NA NA	81.2 76.1[a]	NA NA	21.2 17[a]
β-blockers	13.1 6.9[a]	28 14[a]	84.7 79.9[a]	NA NA	63.4 52.9[a]	NA NA	22 16.8[a]
MRA	NA NA	27 21	23.5 17.2[a]	NA NA	49.8 38[a]	NA NA	16 10[a]

Data presented as percentages (%) unless stated otherwise.

Abbreviations: ACE, angiotensin-converting enzyme; AF, atrial fibrillation; ARBs, angiotensin receptor blockers; BMI, body mass index; CAD, coronary artery disease; COPD, chronic obstructive pulmonary disease; EHFS, EuroHeart Failure Survey; LVEF, left ventricular ejection fraction; MRA, mineralocorticoid receptor antagonist; NA, not applicable; OPTIMIZE-HF, Organized Program to Initiate Lifesaving Treatment in Hospitalized Patients with Heart Failure; PROTECT, Prophylaxis for Thromboembolism in Critical Care; VERITAS trial, Value of Endothelin Receptor Inhibition With Tezosentan in Acute Heart Failure Studies; WMI, wall motion index.

[a] Statistically significant.

[b] Data not available but significantly higher in the elderly.

CLINICAL PRESENTATION OF ELDERLY PATIENTS WITH ACUTE HEART FAILURE

Considerable agreement exists between studies describing the clinical profiles of elderly versus younger patients with AHF. Elderly patients with AHF are predominantly women (60%) and are less commonly obese and diabetic, more commonly hypertensive, and have more often atrial fibrillation compared with younger patients.[6,8,9,11,12,14–16] On the other hand, occurrence of ischemic heart disease is less common in octogenarians than in those younger than 80 years (see **Table 1**; **Table 2**).[6,8,9,11,12,14–16] Recent HF-related medical history is usually less remarkable in elderly patients with AHF. Prior functional capacity graded according to New York Heart Association (NYHA) classification is more commonly better in elderly patients than in their younger counterparts, although this is not a consistent observation across various studies.[7,8,14] Elderly patients are also less likely to have an HF hospitalization in the year before current admission.[14]

New-onset HF is more common in older (45%) than in younger patients (35%) with AHF.[12] Accordingly, rales and elevated jugular venous pressure were reported more commonly in the older than in the younger patients in the Organized Program to Initiate Lifesaving Treatment in Hospitalized Patients with Heart Failure (OPTIMIZE-HF) registry conducted in the United States.[15] Older patients are also more commonly tachypnoic, with lower oxygen saturation on presentation.[8,11,14] Peripheral edema, though, is less likely in the elderly.[15] Initial systolic blood pressure is higher in older patients, although variation exists among different studies depending on the cutoff age defining the elderly.[8,9,12,14,15] Fever or confirmed infection is more common in the elderly, so are atypical symptoms including confusion/decline of cognitive function, appetite loss, and fatigue, which makes differential diagnosis more complex (see **Tables 1** and **2**).[8,12]

Normal or near-normal left ventricular ejection fraction is a more common finding in older versus younger patients, as is left atrial dilatation.[6–9,12,15,16] Regarding laboratory tests, creatinine and serum urea nitrogen levels are higher and estimated glomerular filtration rate is lower in elderly subjects with AHF.[6–8,11,12,16] Serum sodium may also be higher and potassium levels lower in the elderly.[8,16] Levels of natriuretic peptides both on admission and at discharge are higher in the elderly, but variation exists between studies depending on different cutoff ages

---

Table 2
Characteristics of elderly versus younger patients with AHF

	Elderly	Younger
Clinical profile	Women, hypertensive, nonobese, nondiabetic, atrial fibrillation, non-CV comorbidities (stroke, peripheral vascular disease, anemia, frailty)	Men, obese, diabetic, coronary artery disease, less con-CV comorbidities
Clinical presentation	Vascular-type HF Rales, high SBP, increased JVP, low arterial oxygen saturation, infection	Cardiac-type HF Lower SBP, higher peripheral edema, less rales
HF history	New-onset HF No recent HF hospitalization	Acutely decompensated chronic HF Prior HF hospitalization
Laboratory findings	Lower eGFR, higher SUN, higher levels of NPs, lower Hb	Higher eGFR, lower levels of NPs
Echocardiography	Preserved LV systolic function, diastolic dysfunction, LA dilatation	Reduced LV systolic function
Treatment	Lower diuretic doses, less inotropes Less BB, ACEi/ARBs/MRAs	Higher diuretic doses, more inotropes More BB, ACEi/ARBs/MRAs
Highest risk	Tachypnea, low oxygen saturation, CS, high troponin, infection, very elderly, renal dysfunction, frailty	Tachypnea, low oxygen saturation, CS, high troponin, infection, low SBP, diabetes, advanced NYHA, prior HF hospitalization

Abbreviations: ACEi, angiotensin-converting enzyme inhibitor; ARB, angiotensin receptor blockers; BB, β-blocker; CS, cardiogenic shock; CV, cardiovascular; eGFR, estimated glomerular filtration rate; Hb, hemoglobin; JVP, jugular venous pressure; LA, left atrium; LV, left ventricle; MRA, mineralocorticoid receptor antagonists; NP, natriuretic peptide; NYHA, New York Heart Association; SBP, systolic blood pressure; SUN, serum urea nitrogen.

defining elderly.[11,15] Troponin levels are more commonly higher in the elderly.[11,15] Albumin levels are lower in the elderly with AHF, possibly reflecting their worse nutritional status.[11,14]

Table 1 summarizes the main findings of prospective large-scale AHF registries and posthoc analyses of randomized clinical trials comparing elderly with younger patients with AHF.

COMORBIDITIES

Noncardiovascular comorbidities including stroke/transient ischemic attack (TIA), peripheral vascular disease, anemia, and thyroid abnormalities are more common in the elderly than in younger patients with AHF. In most studies, chronic renal impairment is reported more frequently in the elderly, but this varies according to the cutoff age in different studies.[5,7,8,11,12,16] Chronic obstructive pulmonary disease (COPD) is also variably comorbid in elderly patients with AHF, depending on the different definition of the disease in various studies (asthma vs COPD).[6,11,12,14,15] Depression seems more prevalent in older ages. However, owing to limited data and an overlap between depressive symptoms and symptoms related to somatic disabilities, the true prevalence of clinical depression in the elderly may be difficult to estimate.[6,15] Cardiovascular comorbidities occur variably in elderly with AHF. Coronary artery disease and associated risk factors including hyperlipidemia, diabetes, obesity, and smoking habit are more common in younger patients. On the other hand, atrial fibrillation is consistently reported more frequently in the elderly than in younger patients.[11,12,14,15] Arterial hypertension is highly prevalent in all patients with AHF older than 60 years, but it peaks in octogenarians.[14]

Elderly patients with AHF, significantly more frequently than younger patients, have general disabilities, which are due to age-related decline in functional status and which contribute to higher rates of dependency for their everyday self-care and low quality of life. In the EuroHeart Failure Survey (EHFS) II and other studies, elderly compared with younger patients were less likely to live in their own home (87% vs 98%) and more likely to have self-caring problems (59% vs 48%), have walking disorders (80% vs 70%), have difficulties in performing everyday activities (79% vs 72%), and be in need of household assistance from relatives (41% vs 32%) or caring services (28% vs 12%).[12] Thus, elderly with AHF constitute a very frail group of patients who need multidisciplinary approaches in order to improve quality of in-hospital care and to guide postdischarge daily care.[12]

MANAGEMENT OF ELDERLY PATIENTS WITH ACUTE HEART FAILURE

Age-related disparities occur in the management of AHF.[12,15] Elderly patients are less frequently referred for evaluation by a specialist cardiologist in the emergency department compared with younger patients.[8] During their hospitalization, they are about 30% less likely to undergo an echocardiographic evaluation than younger individuals.[8,9,12,15,16] Furthermore, cardiac catheterization and percutaneous coronary artery interventions are less commonly performed in older patients.[9,12]

Intravenous pharmacotherapy of the elderly with AHF includes lower doses of intravenous diuretics, less frequent use of inotropic agents, but similar rates of use of nitrates and vasopressors compared with younger patients.[11,14] Regarding nonpharmacological therapies, noninvasive ventilation is also less commonly used in elderly patients with AHF.[8,11,14]

Differences in the management between older and younger patients with AHF also exist regarding administration of guideline-recommended chronic HF pharmacotherapy during index hospitalization.[18] In the OPTIMIZE-HF registry, angiotensin-converting enzyme (ACE) inhibitors and/or angiotensin receptor blockers (ARBs), β-blockers, and mineralocorticoid receptor antagonists (MRAs) were prescribed less frequently in elderly patients (≥75 years) with HFrEF compared with their younger counterparts.[15] The findings of the EHFS II, as well as of smaller European AHF registries and subanalyses of randomized clinical trials, were similar (see **Table 1**).[9,11,12,14–16,18] On the other hand, digoxin was prescribed more often in the elderly patients in both the OPTIMIZE-HF and the EHFS II.[7,12,14,15] Underprescription of life-saving medications in the elderly could be related to higher rates of comorbidities such as renal dysfunction and of age-related degenerative conditions such as orthostatic hypotension and bradycardia that render elderly patients more often intolerant of neurohormonal antagonists. On the other hand, underprescription of HF drugs may be associated to hospital- or country-level referral policies of elderly patients presenting to emergency departments, resulting in their frequent admission to internal medicine than to cardiology units where physicians may be less familiar with proper initiation and optimal titration of HF medications.[12,14,16] Indeed, in the EHFS II, only 78% of octogenarians admitted with AHF were referred to cardiology departments as opposed to 85% of younger patients.[12] This observation emphasizes the need to disseminate HF guidelines to doctors of cardiology-affiliated specialties, most importantly internal medicine doctors and intesivists, aiming to improve quality of care.

Device implantation is performed in increasing rates in elderly patients. A historical claims-based study from health care databases in the United States showed that 28% of patients eligible for receiving implantable cardioverter-defibrillators (ICD) were octogenarians.[19] In practice, approximately 40% of all patients who receive an ICD are aged 70 years or older, whereas octogenarians constitute approximately 10% of the implanted population.[20] Furthermore, a substantial fraction of elderly patients eligible for receiving cardiac resynchronization therapy-defibrillator (CRT-D) ($\geq$75 years) receive a CRT-D (83%) rather than an ICD (17%).[21] Overall, although both ICD and CRT-D seem to improve survival rates of elderly patients with HF comparable with younger patients, the advantage of sudden death prevention by devices may be attenuated by the higher nonarrhythmic mortality in older age groups.[22,23] Therefore, device therapy should be reserved for highly selected patients at high risk of arrhythmic death and with few comorbidities, with an expected life expectancy of greater than 5 to 7 years, in order for these therapies to be cost effective.[24]

OUTCOMES OF ELDERLY PATIENTS WITH ACUTE HEART FAILURE

Outcomes of elderly patients hospitalized for AHF are significantly worse than those of younger subjects, in terms of in-hospital, short- and long-term mortality. More specifically, in the OPTIMIZE-HF registry, elderly patients ($\geq$75 years), as compared with their younger counterparts, had double rates of in-hospital mortality (4.9% vs 2.4%, $P<.001$) and 1.5 times higher postdischarge short-term mortality (12.76% vs 8.11%, $P<.001$).[15] In the Prophylaxis for Thromboembolism in Critical Care (PROTECT) trial, the 6-month mortality in octogenarians was double than that of patients younger than 80 years (23.9% vs 11.3%, $P<.001$). Each 5-year increase in age resulted in 17% increase in the mortality risk.[14] Similarly, in a Danish multicenter study of hospitalized HF patients, advancing age (per 10-year increase of age) was independently associated with 23% increase in 30-day mortality risk and 55% increase in 5- to 8-year mortality risk.[7]

Data regarding rehospitalizations in older versus younger patients with AHF are less consistent across various studies. In the EHFS II, younger patients had approximately 30% higher risk of rehospitalization from discharge to 3 months after and from 3 to 9 months postdischarge.[12] On the other hand, the VERITAS (Value of Endothelin Receptor Inhibition With Tezosentan in Acute Heart Failure Studies) trial reported higher rates of 30-day rehospitalization in older versus younger patients (8.1% vs 6.7%).[11] No significant differences in rehospitalization rates were reported in the OPTIMIZE-HF registry at 2 to 3 months after hospital discharge and in the PROTECT trial from discharge to 7 days after between older and younger patients.[14,15] Moreover, a large-scale single-center retrospective study of approximately 9500 patients with AHF reported similar annualized rates of total and HF-related readmissions but 20% higher annualized rate of non-HF readmissions in patients aged 75 years or older compared with patients younger than 75 years.[6]

Reports of LOS of elderly versus younger patients with AHF vary.[11,15,25] No significant difference was observed between LOS of elderly ($\geq$75 years) versus younger patients in the North American OPTIMIZE-HF registry, where the mean LOS was 5.6 versus 5.8 days for the elderly and younger patients, respectively.[15] On the contrary, in the VERITAS trial, younger patients had a shorter LOS than older patients by a mean of 1.15 days.[11]

PREDICTORS OF CLINICAL OUTCOMES OF ELDERLY PATIENTS WITH ACUTE HEART FAILURE

Parameters indicating a severe initial presentation (tachypnea, low arterial blood oxygen saturation, cardiogenic shock, troponin elevation, acute infection) are associated with worse in-hospital and short-term postdischarge outcomes in both elderly and younger patients with AHF.[8,12,14] However, a differential effect of systolic blood pressure on short-term outcomes of elderly versus younger patients is reported. In elderly patients aged 75 years and older, the favorable effect of higher systolic blood pressure on presentation, which is seen in patients of age less than 75 years, is attenuated.[11,14] Furthermore, differences exist regarding the association of historical factors with short-term outcomes of older versus younger patients. Age itself, a history of COPD, diabetes, chronic renal impairment, valvular heart disease, and severe age-related disabilities such as bed confinement predict worse outcomes in the elderly. On the other hand, short-term outcomes of younger patients is not influenced by comorbidities, except for diabetes mellitus.[11] Also, prior severely limited functional status (NYHA class IV) and recent HF hospitalization are associated with unfavorable outcomes only in younger patients,

Table 3
Summary of differences and similarities of AHF in elderly patients between the European EHFS II and the North American OPTIMIZE-HF registries

	OPTIMIZE-HF		EHFS II	
Date	2003–2004		2004–2005	
Centers	259 hospitals/United States		133 hospitals/30 ESC countries	
Patients, n	48,612		3577	
Mean age, y	73.2		71.5	
Age cutoff (y); %	<75; 47.2	≥75; 52.8	<80; 79	≥80; 21
Male, %	56.2	41.1*	66	44*
BMI or weight in kg	90.2 kg	71.2 kg*	26.9	26*
Creatinine, mg/dL	1.6	1.9*	1.2	1.3*
CAD, %	43.7	47.5*	54	51
AF, %	21.7	39*	36	48*
Hypertension, %	71.9	70.1*	61	67*
Diabetes, %	27.3	22.8*	34	29
COPD, %	27.4	27.8	19	22*
Depression, %	11.3	10.1	57	55
Hemoglobin, g/dL	12.3	12*	12.5	13*
Echo performed, %	88.4	84.8*	92	81*
Coronary angiography reported, %	17	41*	NA	NA
Percutaneous intervention performed, %	5	9*	NA	NA
HFpEF, %	40.8	55.3*	28	39*
LVEF cutoff, %	≥40		≥45%	
ACE inhibitors/ARBs, %	84.3	78.8*	81.2	76.1*
β-blockers, %	84.7	79.9*	63.4	52.9*
MRAs, %	23.5	17.2*	49.8	38*
Median LOS (IQR), d	4 (2–7)	4 (3–7)[a]	NA	NA
In-hospital mortality, %	2.4	4.9*	5.6	10.7*
3-mo postdischarge mortality, %	8.1	12.8*	6.8	13.5*
3-mo rehospitalization rates, %	29.8	29.4	NA	

Abbreviations: AF, atrial fibrillation; BMI, body mass index; CAD, coronary artery disease; ESC, european society of cardiology; IQR, interquartile range; NA, not available.

* $P<.05$ in older vs younger patients.

[a] Unadjusted $P<.001$; $P = .734$ after adjustment for multivariate prognostic factors.

whereas their prognostic effect is attenuated in elderly patients with AHF.[8,14] The above-mentioned differences of prognosticators between elderly and younger patients with AHF may be related to the different clinical profiles of these 2 subgroups, with elderly patients having a higher prevalence of vascular-type, hypertensive, new-onset AHF with preserved LV systolic function compared with younger individuals.[26] In support of this explanation are the findings of a previously published meta-analysis of 39,372 patients with chronic HF, which showed that systolic blood pressure is less predictive of mortality in patients with HFpEF than in those with HFrEF.[27]

Among laboratory parameters, low serum sodium levels, low serum albumin levels, and high troponin levels are all associated with worse short-term outcomes in both the elderly and younger patients with AHF (see **Table 2**).[11,14] On the other hand, anemia is independently associated with worse short-term outcomes in elderly patients, whereas in the long-term, it confers a higher risk in younger patients with AHF, in whom it may reflect, in addition to neurohormonal and inflammatory activation, the role of hemodilution and thus fluid retention.[11,28]

Long-term prognosis of elderly patients with AHF is largely defined by multimorbidity and disabilities contributing to self-care problems.[12] Furthermore, prescription of ACE inhibitors/ARBs and statins were associated with better long-term outcomes of octogenarians with AHF in the EHFS II.[12] In comparison, advanced NYHA class and previous HF hospitalization and, among comorbidities, diabetes mellitus, are independent negative prognosticators of the long-term outcomes of younger patients with AHF in several studies.[6,9,11,14,16]

COMPARISON OF THE EUROPEAN AND NORTH AMERICAN EXPERIENCE IN ELDERLY WITH ACUTE HEART FAILURE

A comparison of the EHFS II and the OPTIMIZE-HF registry provides a view of similarities and differences of AHF affecting elderly individuals in Europe and the United States, respectively (**Table 3**).[12,15] In the EHFS, the cut point defining elderly patients was 80 years, whereas in the US registry, the respective age was 75 years. Female preponderance; rates of various comorbidities including arterial hypertension, diabetes, and COPD; and prescription of ACE inhibitors/ARBs are similar between the European and American elderly subjects with AHF. Differences are observed in the rates of atrial fibrillation in the elderly (39% in Europe vs 48% in the United States), as well as in the prescription of β-blockers, which are underprescribed in European countries (52.9% in Europe vs 79.9% in the United States), and MRAs, which are prescribed less in the United States (38% in Europe vs 17.2% in the United States). Underprescription of all guideline-recommended neurohormonal antagonists in elderly patients versus their younger counterparts is observed in both sides of the Atlantic. Furthermore, diagnostic modalities (such as echocardiography) and other nonpharmacological interventions (smoking cessation counseling) are similarly underused in elderly versus younger patients in both Europe and the United States. Increasing trends in the prescription of guideline-recommended HF drugs in hospitalized octogenarians with AHF are reported in the European countries, as shown by the comparison of the EHFS I (conducted between 2000 and 2001) and II (conducted between 2004 and 2005). In EHFS II versus I there was an increase in rates of prescription of ACE inhibitors/ARBs (76.1% from 56%), β-blockers (53% from 25%), and MRAs (38% from 15%).[12,29] A trend for dose uptitration of life-saving medications in octogenarians is also observed in European countries from 2000 to 2005.[12,29] Similar trends in the prescription of neurohormonal antagonists in the elderly have

been observed in the United States, according to registries conducted from 2002 to 2004.[10] The improvements of implementation of HF drug therapies have resulted from ongoing, widespread dissemination of international guidelines coupled with the increasing enrollment of patients in dedicated disease management programs.

Clinical outcomes of elderly patients with AHF may vary between Europe and the United States. In-hospital mortality in octogenarians with AHF was more than double in European countries compared with that in the United States (10.7% vs 4.9%). Furthermore, the 2- to 3-month mortality postdischarge was 12.76% in the United States, close to the reported rate in Europe (13.5%). However, variation may exist between Europe and the United States regarding LOS of elderly patients with AHF. In the OPTIMIZE-HF, the median LOS of elderly AHF patients was 4 days, whereas in the Western European cohort of patients with AHF enrolled in the PROTECT trial, the median LOS of the entire cohort (older and younger patients) was 10 days.[4,15]

SUMMARY AND FUTURE DIRECTIONS

So far, the elderly AHF population has been underrepresented in large-scale trials of newly tested drugs, owing to safety concerns that result from higher rates of renal and liver dysfunction in the elderly, which are common routes of excretion of various drugs. Pharmacokinetics of investigational drugs may be altered because of the lower body mass, fat tissue, and total body water content of this population. In the future, elderly and very elderly patients should be enrolled in all new pharmaceutical trials, targeting a more real-world population. Apart from inclusion criteria, monitoring of outcomes and treatment goals have to be appropriately adjusted when including elderly patients.

Data show that elderly patients with AHF may not be admitted to cardiology units but rather to internal medicine and geriatric departments or intensive care units, where treating physicians are usually internal medicine doctors and intensivists.[12,14,16] Health care providers will have to intensify educational programs aiming to disseminate international HF guidelines to include doctors of other specialties, in order to improve quality of care of the elderly with AHF. Furthermore, as shown in large-scale European registries, prescription rates of HF life-saving medications in the elderly increase during hospitalization but remain stable after discharge.[12] Therefore, every effort should be undertaken to initiate and optimize guideline-recommended HF medications while the patients are still hospitalized.

Specific attention should be paid to the HFpEF subgroup, which is prevalent among elderly patients with AHF. Echocardiography has to be prioritized in all patients with AHF to identify the subcategory of HF. The prognostic effect of standard structural and functional cardiac abnormalities, together with novel measurements of systolic dysfunction including global longitudinal strain in HFpEF, should be appropriately defined in well-designed prospective studies. Moreover, pharmaceutical research should set a priority in developing and evaluating new pharmacologic agents that would specifically target HFpEF, including elderly patients in future studies. At present, serelaxin, a natural vasodilator, is being tested in phase 3 trials for the treatment of patients with AHF irrespective of the ejection fraction.[30] Likewise, new medications including soluble guanylate cyclase stimulators and neprilysin inhibitors are being tested in phase 2b and 3 trials, respectively, for their effectiveness in patients with chronic HFpEF.

Finally, frailty of elderly patients should be taken under consideration when defining the individual therapeutic strategy. A holistic approach and palliative care may be recommended in cases with a poor outlook. Planned and ongoing global HF registries are expected to shed more light on current challenges and limitations of medical management of this distinct HF population.

REFERENCES

1. Mozaffarian D, Benjamin EJ, Go AS, et al. Heart disease and stroke statistics–2015 update: a report from the American Heart Association. Circulation 2015;131(4):e29–322.

2. Andersson C, Vasan RS. Epidemiology of heart failure with preserved ejection fraction. Heart Fail Clin 2014;10(3):377–88.

3. Kumar R, Gandhi SK, Little WC. Acute heart failure with preserved systolic function. Crit Care Med 2008;36(1 Suppl):S52–6.

4. Mentz RJ, Cotter G, Cleland JG, et al. International differences in clinical characteristics, management, and outcomes in acute heart failure patients: better short-term outcomes in patients enrolled in Eastern Europe and Russia in the PROTECT trial. Eur J Heart Fail 2014;16(6):614–24.

5. Mogensen UM, Ersboll M, Andersen M, et al. Clinical characteristics and major comorbidities in heart failure patients more than 85 years of age compared with younger age groups. Eur J Heart Fail 2011; 13(11):1216–23.

6. Stein GY, Kremer A, Shochat T, et al. The diversity of heart failure in a hospitalized population: the role of age. J Card Fail 2012;18(8):645–53.

7. Gustafsson F, Torp-Pedersen C, Seibaek M, et al. Effect of age on short and long-term mortality in patients admitted to hospital with congestive heart failure. Eur Heart J 2004;25(19):1711–7.

8. Herrero-Puente P, Martin-Sanchez FJ, Fernandez-Fernandez M, et al. Differential clinical characteristics and outcome predictors of acute heart failure in elderly patients. Int J Cardiol 2012;155(1):81–6.

9. Pulignano G, Del Sindaco D, Tavazzi L, et al. Clinical features and outcomes of elderly outpatients with heart failure followed up in hospital cardiology units: data from a large nationwide cardiology database (IN-CHF Registry). Am Heart J 2002; 143(1):45–55.

10. Fonarow GC, Heywood JT, Heidenreich PA, et al. Temporal trends in clinical characteristics, treatments, and outcomes for heart failure hospitalizations, 2002 to 2004: findings from Acute Decompensated Heart Failure National Registry (ADHERE). Am Heart J 2007;153(6):1021–8.

11. Metra M, Cotter G, El-Khorazaty J, et al. Acute heart failure in the elderly: differences in clinical characteristics, outcomes, and prognostic factors in the VERITAS Study. J Card Fail 2015;21(3):179–88.

12. Komajda M, Hanon O, Hochadel M, et al. Contemporary management of octogenarians hospitalized for heart failure in Europe: Euro Heart Failure Survey II. Eur Heart J 2009;30(4):478–86.

13. Follath F, Yilmaz MB, Delgado JF, et al. Clinical presentation, management and outcomes in the Acute Heart Failure Global Survey of Standard Treatment (ALARM-HF). Intensive Care Med 2011;37(4):619–26.

14. Metra M, Mentz RJ, Chiswell K, et al. Acute heart failure in elderly patients: worse outcomes and differential utility of standard prognostic variables. Insights from the PROTECT trial. Eur J Heart Fail 2015;17(1):109–18.

15. Fonarow GC, Abraham WT, Albert NM, et al. Age- and gender-related differences in quality of care and outcomes of patients hospitalized with heart failure (from OPTIMIZE-HF). Am J Cardiol 2009;104(1):107–15.

16. Mahjoub H, Rusinaru D, Souliere V, et al. Long-term survival in patients older than 80 years hospitalised for heart failure. A 5-year prospective study. Eur J Heart Fail 2008;10(1):78–84.

17. Rich MW. Management of heart failure in the elderly. Heart Fail Rev 2002;7(1):89–97.

18. Gislason GH, Rasmussen JN, Abildstrom SZ, et al. Persistent use of evidence-based pharmacotherapy in heart failure is associated with improved outcomes. Circulation 2007;116(7):737–44.

19. Ruskin JN, Camm AJ, Zipes DP, et al. Implantable cardioverter defibrillator utilization based on discharge diagnoses from Medicare and managed

care patients. J Cardiovasc Electrophysiol 2002; 13(1):38–43.

20. Barra S, Providencia R, Paiva L, et al. Implantable cardioverter-defibrillators in the elderly: rationale and specific age-related considerations. Europace 2015;17(2):174–86.

21. Heidenreich PA, Tsai V, Bao H, et al. Does Age Influence Cardiac Resynchronization Therapy Use and Outcome? JACC Heart Fail 2015;3(6):497–504.

22. Huang DT, Sesselberg HW, McNitt S, et al. Improved survival associated with prophylactic implantable defibrillators in elderly patients with prior myocardial infarction and depressed ventricular function: a MADIT-II substudy. J Cardiovasc Electrophysiol 2007;18(8):833–8.

23. Chan PS, Nallamothu BK, Spertus JA, et al. Impact of age and medical comorbidity on the effectiveness of implantable cardioverter-defibrillators for primary prevention. Circ Cardiovasc Qual Outcomes 2009; 2(1):16–24.

24. Connolly SJ, Hallstrom AP, Cappato R, et al. Meta-analysis of the implantable cardioverter defibrillator secondary prevention trials. AVID, CASH and CIDS studies. Antiarrhythmics vs implantable defibrillator study. cardiac arrest study hamburg.

canadian implantable defibrillator study. Eur Heart J 2000;21(24):2071–8.

25. Ezekowitz JA, Bakal JA, Kaul P, et al. Acute heart failure in the emergency department: short and long-term outcomes of elderly patients with heart failure. Eur J Heart Fail 2008;10(3):308–14.

26. Lazzarini V, Mentz RJ, Fiuzat M, et al. Heart failure in elderly patients: distinctive features and unresolved issues. Eur J Heart Fail 2013;15(7):717–23.

27. Pocock SJ, Ariti CA, McMurray JJ, et al. Predicting survival in heart failure: a risk score based on 39 372 patients from 30 studies. Eur Heart J 2013; 34(19):1404–13.

28. van der Meer P, Postmus D, Ponikowski P, et al. The predictive value of short-term changes in hemoglobin concentration in patients presenting with acute decompensated heart failure. J Am Coll Cardiol 2013;61(19):1973–81.

29. Komajda M, Hanon O, Hochadel M, et al. Management of octogenarians hospitalized for heart failure in Euro Heart Failure Survey I. Eur Heart J 2007; 28(11):1310–8.

30. Filippatos G, Teerlink JR, Farmakis D, et al. Serelaxin in acute heart failure patients with preserved left ventricular ejection fraction: results from the RELAX-AHF trial. Eur Heart J 2014;35(16):1041–50.

Characteristics of Intensive Care in Patients Hospitalized for Heart Failure in Europe

Ovidiu Chioncel, MD, PhD, FHFA[a],*,
Alexandre Mebazaa, MD, FESC, FHFA[b]

KEYWORDS

- Acute heart failure • Cardiac intensive care • Therapies

KEY POINTS

- Intensive care unit (ICU) it is a high-technology, life-saving care environment that provides advanced care to the sickest heart failure patients.
- Information provided by contemporary heart failure (HF) registries suggests that ICU admission rates differ considerably across Europe.
- A considerably higher utilization of intravenous (IV) therapies and interventional procedures was typically found in ICU departments.
- The subgroup of acute HF (AHF) patients managed in ICUs had the highest rate of in-hospital mortality compared with the rest of the care settings.

INTRODUCTION

Acute heart failure (AHF) is a complex syndrome with heterogeneous clinical presentations requiring urgent therapies.[1] Despite hospitalization, AHF patients remain at substantial risk of in-hospital and postdischarge mortality.[1,2] AHF patients are diagnosed and managed in a diversity of medical care settings, including emergency departments (EDs), cardiology departments, and intensive care units (ICUs).

Patients hospitalized for AHF may clinically decompensate and experience life-threatening complications that require immediate supportive therapies available only in an ICU. Although there are large variations in definition, ICU offers a high-technology, life-saving care environment that supports any isolated or combined advanced organ dysfunction. Distinct to coronary care units (CCUs), which generally admit patients with isolated cardiac dysfunction, mostly myocardial infarction patients or HF patients,[3] ICUs may admit the most severe AHF patients with as high an index of clinical and biological severity as those with cardiogenic shock (CS) or those requiring advanced respiratory support or support for multiple organ failure.[4] Furthermore, ICUs are

Disclosure Statement: O. Chioncel has nothing to disclose; A. Mebazaa received speaker's honoraria from The Medicines Company, Novartis, Orion, Roche, and Servier; A. Mebazaa received fee as member of advisory board and/or Steering Committee from Cardiorentis, The Medicine Company, Adrenomed, MyCartis, ZS Pharma, and Critical Diagnostics.
[a] ICCU and Cardiology 1st Department, Institute of Emergency for Cardiovascular Diseases "C.C.Iliescu", University of Medicine Carol Davila, sos Fundeni, no 258, Bucharest sect 2, Romania; [b] Department of Anesthesia and Critical Care, Hôpital Lariboisière, DAR, Hôpitaux Universitaires Saint Louis Lariboisière, APHP, University Paris Diderot, 2 Rue A Paré, Paris Cedex 10 75475, France
* Corresponding author.
E-mail address: ochioncel@yahoo.co.uk

Heart Failure Clin 11 (2015) 647–656
http://dx.doi.org/10.1016/j.hfc.2015.07.005
1551-7136/15/$ — see front matter © 2015 Elsevier Inc. All rights reserved.

characterized by high-intensity staffing in terms of nurse and physician–to-patient ratio.[4]

Some AHF patients are in critical condition early at presentation, admitted directly to an ICU, whereas other AHF patients may aggravate sometime during hospitalization and need ICU care. Regardless of the timing of ICU transfer and despite innovations of high-technology organ support[5,6] and improving clinical expertise and practice staffing[7,8] of physicians attending critically ill patients, the ICU setting admits HF patients at increased risk of in-hospital mortality.[9–11]

This articles describes, from the European perspective, clinical characteristics, management patterns, and in-hospital outcomes of AHF patients managed in ICU departments.

DATA SOURCE INFORMATION

There is limited information about epidemiology and outcome of AHF patients admitted to ICU departments, and these data are provided by analysis of national or continental administrative data,[12,13] observational studies and registries,[9–11] and randomized clinical trials.[14] Furthermore, the diversity of health care structures and policies[12] and differing nomenclature used throughout Europe can lead to confusion when describing ICU/CCU care and make it difficult to examine this care setting in AHF patients.

Even if analysis of administrative data resulted from national health statistics and hospital discharge records offer information related to health care expenditure, number of ICU beds, number of hospitalizations, and related cost, these data do not capture information related to initial clinical presentation and cannot be used to evaluate clinical probability of ICU admission.

Distinct to administrative data, observational studies and registries offer extensive information about clinical, management, and outcome characteristics of real-life AHF patients prior to ICU admission and during whole hospitalization. Although a majority of contemporary European HF registries reported ICU or CCU admission rates, only 2 of

them, the Romanian Acute Heart Failure Syndromes (RO-AHFS) registry[9] and the Acute Heart Failure Global Survey of Standard Treatment (ALARM-HF)[11] provided post hoc analysis focused on AHF patients admitted to an ICU. Additional information was provided by the French national study, EFICA, (Etude Française de l'Insuffisance Cardiaque Aiguë)[10] describing a mixed population admitted to both ICU and CCU departments.

Randomized controlled trials provide valuable epidemiologic data, but the applicability of this information is limited by the fact that clinical trials use selective inclusion and exclusion criteria to focus on a specific subgroup of patients and report less severe cardiac and noncardiac comorbidities, and, consequently, a lower event rate. Regional differences in baseline characteristics, in-hospital management, and postdischarge outcome for AHF patients requiring CCU and ICU level care have been recently reported in the Acute Study of Clinical Effectiveness of Nesiritide in Decompensated Heart Failure (ASCEND-HF) trial.[14] Data from AHF patients enrolled in Europe are included in this article.

INTENSIVE CARE UNIT ADMISSION RATES

Generally, reported ICU admission rates in AHF registries[9,11,15–19] varied according to methodology and local practices of the studies, but description overall is poor, because most of the studies reported a cumulative rate in both ICUs and CCUs (Table 1). If cumulative rate is similar in most of the HF registries, specific ICU admission rates varied considerably, from 45.4% reported in ALARM-HF study[11] to 5% in the recent Observatoire Française de l'Insuffisance Cardiaque Aigue (OFICA) survey.[17]

Wide national variations regarding ICU bed capacity may contribute to these regional differences.[12,13] Recent European statistics reported that the overall number of ICU beds across European countries varied between 3.5 and 21.9 per 100,000 inhabitants, and similar large variations were noted when ICU beds were reported to total bed capacity, 1.2 to 4.4 ICU beds per 100 hospital beds. ICU bed capacity did not parallel national

Table 1 ICU admission rate in different European registries						
	EHFS II[16]	FIN-AKVA[15]	OFICA[17]	ALARM-HF[9]	IN HF[18]	RO-AHFS[11]
ICU (%)	—	11.9	5	45	—	10.7
Cumulative ICU/CCU (%)	51	51.4	40	74.8	51.9	71.3
LOS ICU (d)	3	2	—	4		4

Abbreviations: ALARM-HF, Acute Heart Failure Global Survey of Standard treatment; EHFS II- EuroHeart Failure Survey II; FIN-AKVA, Finish Acute Heart Failure Study; IN HF, Italian Registry on Heart Failure Outcome; LOS, length of stay; OFICA, Observatoire Française de l'Insuffisance Cardiaque Aigue; RO-AHFS- Romanian Acute Heart Failure Syndromes registry.

health expenditure, suggesting that health care models in each country have a major impact on the development and prioritization of this resource.[12] The decision to transfer patients to an ICU, however, is influenced by a combination of factors, including patient severity, ICU availability, medical staff experience, and local protocols.

Also, the paucity of guideline recommendations regarding ICU triage[1] leaves disposition decision making to the discretion of individual providers and likely contributes to the observed geographic variability. A recent consensus article[20] provides practical recommendation for ICU admission in high-risk AHF patients.

Initial clinical presentation did have an impact on rate of ICU admission and patients presenting with more severe clinical profiles, because CS and pulmonary edema are more frequently referred to ICU.[9–11]

Although the most severe AHF patients are admitted to an ICU, the specific medical reason for ICU admission and the type of ICU admission (direct admission from ED or transfer during hospitalization) were not commonly collected by European registries. In the RO-AHFS registry, the most common reason for ICU transfers was the need for mechanical ventilatory support (31%), followed by management of complex vasoactive infusions (25%), post–cardiopulmonary resuscitation (19%), and worsening of associated noncardiac comorbidities (17%). Only one-third of these patients were admitted directly to the ICU from the ED and a majority of patients were transferred to the ICU sometime after admission, suggesting ongoing clinical decompensation despite hospitalization. The findings support recent recommendations, which suggest that the medical decision for triage to the ICU setting is generally best accomplished based on specific findings that require intensive monitoring and therapy for compromised respiratory or hemodynamic status.[20]

BASELINE CHARACTERISTICS OF PATIENTS ADMITTED TO INTENSIVE CARE UNITS

At initial presentation, compared with patients treated in usual care, ICU patients had lower systolic blood pressure (SBP) and higher heart rate and respiratory rate (RR), suggesting marked neurohormonal activation.[9–11] In ALARM-HF,[11] a proportion of 27.7% of patients admitted to ICUs had SBP less than 100 mm Hg, and in the RO-AHFS registry,[9] 53% had SBP less than 110 mm Hg. The proportion of patients with CS was higher in ICU departments compared with CCUs or wards (**Fig. 1**). In the EFICA study, including a mixed ICU and CCU population, 29% of patients had CS.[10]

Echocardiography was available in approximately 80% of patients admitted to critical care departments.[9–11] A majority of AHF patients who required ICU care had left ventricular systolic dysfunction. The proportion of patients with HF with preserved ejection fraction was 20.6% in the RO-AHFS study[9] and 27% in EFICA,[10] demonstrating that AHF event with relatively preserved systolic function can be severe enough to require intensive care interventions.

Patients managed in ICUs had a high incidence of arrhythmias that may be explained by the underlying condition being treated or concomitant therapies that are arrhythmogenic.[9,10]

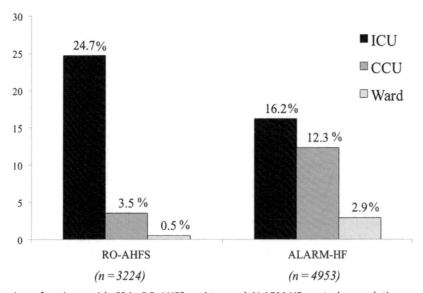

Fig. 1. Proportion of patients with CS in RO-AHFS registry and ALARM-HF. *n*, study population.

Organ dysfunction was common in AHF patients admitted to ICU/CCU departments. In the EFICA study,[10] 53% of patients had renal dysfunction and 61% had liver dysfunction. Renal dysfunction can be explained by high rates of comorbid conditions, such as hypertension and diabetes, and by hemodynamic abnormalities, including high venous pressure and low blood flow. Hepatic dysfunction is associated with a constellation of clinical findings suggestive of abnormal hemodynamics including venous congestion and poor end-organ perfusion. In a previous subgroup analysis of the RO-AHFS study,[21] higher alanine aminotransferase at admission was independently predictive of in-hospital outcomes including necessity for ICU admission.

Hyponatremia observed in ICU patients can be the result of neurohormonal activation, including stimulation of vassopresin, and additionally can be produced by several noncardiac comorbidities, such as pneumonia, cirrhosis, and hypothyroidism.[22]

IN-HOSPITAL THERAPIES AND INVASIVE PROCEDURES

The utilization of IV therapies and procedural interventions in HF patients receiving ICU/CCU-level care is higher, but few large observational experiences in this high-acuity population have been conducted to date.

Utilization of IV inotropes was substantially higher among patients managed in ICUs (**Fig. 2**), and 53% of patients enrolled in EFICA study[10] and 56.7% of ICU patients in RO-AHFS registry[9] were treated with IV inotropes.

Among European countries participating in the ALARM-HF, utilization of IV inotropes varied between 26% and 47%, reflecting differences in local and regional pattern of care as well as different levels of medical expertise.

Utilization of IV inotropes in CCU departments was lower in the RO-AHFS registry compared with ALARM-HF (see **Fig. 2**). This pattern, as well as lower proportion of patients with CS managed in CCUs (see **Fig. 1**), suggests a lower threshold for ICU admission or inferior performance of CCU departments in Romanian hospitals.

Vasopressors were almost exclusively used in the ICU setting and are added in patients who remain hypotensive despite adequate fluid replacement and despite up-titrating of inotropic therapy. Decreasing of systemic vascular resistance in ICU setting can be caused by either systemic inflammatory response syndrome, sepsis, or alternatively severe hemodynamic compromise with occurrence of multiple organ failure.[23]

In the RO-AHFS and ALARM registries, use of inotropes does not seem to follow recent recommendations.[20] IV inotropes were administrated to a high proportion of patients with SBP greater than 110 mm Hg at initial clinical presentation. This may also indicate that, in at least a subset of AHF patients, clinical stability may worsen as a result of progressive deterioration or secondary to other IV therapies (ie, aggressive loop diuretics and/or vasodilators).

Invasive interventions and procedures are predominantly, or, for some of them, exclusively used in ICU departments (**Table 2**), a finding explained by organization of medical care in European countries, variation in the availability of resources among participating sites, and, to some extent, by performance of cardiology departments included in the registries. In the RO-AHFS study,[9] 32.7% of ICU patients required invasive mechanical ventilation (IMV) compared with 35% in the EFICA study[10] and 30% in ALARM-HF.[11]

In many European countries, ICU is the only authorized place to offer mechanical ventilation, either invasive or noninvasive, a feature distinct to participating hospitals from ALARM-HF, where mechanical ventilation was performed even on wards (see **Table 2**).

Even if mechanical ventilation is a life-saving therapy in the care of critically ill patients, it is associated with immediate deleterious cardiac effects, such as decrease in cardiac output and SBP, and in-hospital complications, such as barotrauma, respiratory, and systemic infections.[24,25]

Geographic differences in use of IV therapies and procedures have been also found in clinical trials enrolling AHF patients in different care settings, including CCUs.[14] Although, the rates of IV therapies and procedures are lower than those reported by observational studies (**Fig. 3**A), analysis of the clinical trials data may provide a more organized perspective to explore regional differences in utilization of critical care departments for AHF patients. In ASCEND-HF,[14] worldwide differences in the in-hospital pharmacologic treatments and the application of mechanical technologies and cardiac procedures were observed among AHF patients admitted to CCUs. In Europe, a lower proportion (14.4%) of AHF patients were treated with IV inotropes during their CCU stay, compared with Asia Pacific (21.7%) and North America (18.1%). Approximately 11% of all Asian-Pacific, Latin American, and North American patients underwent mechanical ventilation compared with 2.3% of patients enrolled in Europe. Furthermore, use of other invasive procedures or mechanical therapies was lowest in European countries

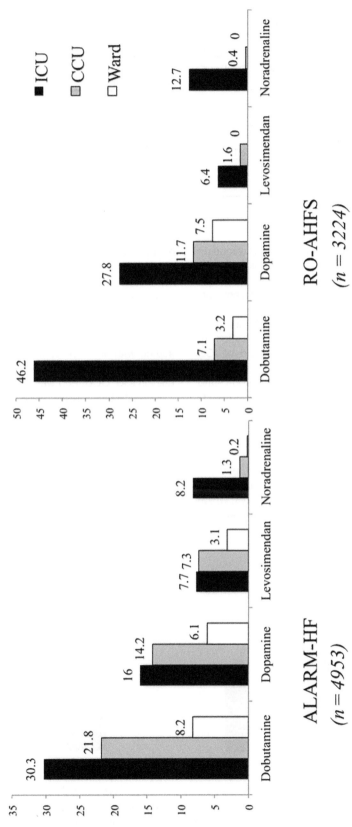

Fig. 2. Rate (%) of utilization of IV inotropes and vasopressors in different care settings; data from RO-AHFS and ALARM-HF registries. *n*, study population.

Table 2
Mechanical therapies by type of care settings

	RO-AHFS Registry[9]			ALARM-HF[11]		
	Intensive Care Unit	Cardiac Care Unit	Ward	Intensive Care Unit	Cardiac Care Unit	Ward
IMV (%)	32.7	0	0	30.0	6.8	2.3
NIMV (%)	6.3	0	0	15.8	6.3	2.2
IABP (%)	2.1	0	0	6.1	6.6	0.4
Pacemaker (%)	4.3	2.1	0.9	3.2	2.4	1.1
Cardioversion (%)	12.4	5.8	3.9	9.5	6.4	6.3
Ultrafiltration (%)	9.4	0	0	—	—	—

Data from RO-AHFS registry and ALARM-HF.
Abbreviations: IABP, intra-aortic balloon pump; NIMV, noninvasive mechanical ventilation.

compared with the other regions.[14] This suggests the existence of the possible geographic variation in level of facilities available in CCUs, different thresholds for CCU admission, and different patterns of enrollment in clinical trials.

In some European registries,[9,11] ICU stay was associated with lower in-hospital utilization of evidence-based HF therapies. A period of ICU admission places HF patients at higher risk for potential discontinuation of their medications, and the transition period after ICU admission is generally too short for initiation of the medications.

INTENSIVE CARE UNIT OUTCOMES

In contemporary European registries, patients admitted and treated in ICU departments had a median length of stay in an ICU of 4 days, which contributed to a longer total duration of hospitalization compared with patients who never stayed in an ICU.[9–11]

In the same registries, patients managed in ICUs had a high rate of all-cause mortality (ACM), a finding not surprising in a subgroup of AHF patients with a high index of clinical and biological severity who require immediate supportive therapies in a setting with high risk of iatrogenic complications. Furthermore, there was a graded in-hospital mortality in ICU, CCU, and ward patients (**Fig. 4**).

As related to postdischarge mortality, the EFICA study reported a 30-day ACM of 27.4% and 1-year ACM of 46.5%, suggesting that the risk of death extends beyond the period of hospitalization, and a CCU/ICU admission is associated with short-term increase in mortality. Although with lower postdischarge mortality values (see **Fig. 3**B) specific to randomized clinical trial setting, a similar trend has been reported by ASCEND-HF[14] in European

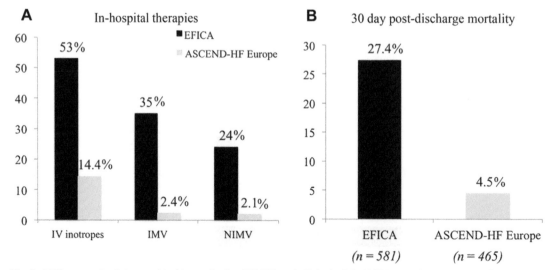

Fig. 3. Differences in data provided by registries (EFICA) and clinical trials (ASCEND-HF). Comparison between in-hospital therapies (*A*) and 30-day mortality (*B*). n, study population; NIMV, noninvasive mechanical ventilation.

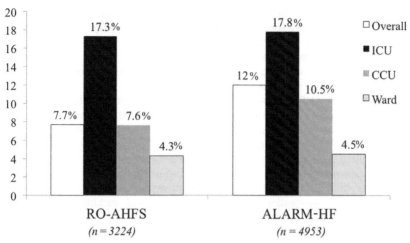

Fig. 4. In-hospital all-cause mortality in ICU, CCU, and ward. Data from RO-AHFS and ALARM-HF registries. *n*, study population.

patients, demonstrating a stepwise increase in mortality between 30 days and 180 days postdischarge (4.5%–11%). In the same trial, despite wide variations in treatment practices, no regional international differences in 30-day all-cause death were observed, suggesting that high-risk characteristics of AHF patients admitted to critical care areas, rather than geographic variation in intensity of therapies, may be the principal determinant of prognosis in this higher-risk subset of patients. Furthermore, even after adjustment for clinical relevant covariates, a critical care admission for AHF was an independent negative prognostic marker.

In the RO-AHFS registry, a direct ICU admission strategy was associated with lower in-hospital ACM and shorter hospitalization, suggesting that triaging patients to the appropriate level of care at presentation can potentially result in improvements in the quality of care and outcomes of patients hospitalized with AHF. Also, higher mortality rates observed in ICU patients transferred sometime after admission suggested that some at-risk patients could be admitted to an ICU at an earlier stage of severity, and their outcome would have been improved. This implies that an unmet clinical need is identifying those patients with occult disease earlier, prior to occurrence of a life-threatening complication on the floor, avoiding transferring them in extremis in ICU. Finding a middle ground is important, however, because overuse of this strategy increases ICU admission rates and consumption of limited physical and financial resources.

INTENSIVE CARE UNIT TRIAGE

To provide appropriate care, critically ill AHF patients need to be identified and managed expertly in a suitable location. Appropriate use of intensive care resources is of fundamental importance because of expensive costs associated with ICU stay and universal shortage of ICU beds. On the other hand, a delay in admission to the ICU may result in a delay in definitive care that is crucial to the outcome of high-risk patients.[26] Application of a risk-prediction algorithm at presentation may identify HF patients more likely to derive a robust benefit from direct ICU admission, and aggressive monitoring and intervention and may aid in avoiding unnecessary ICU admissions.[27] This is crucial in conditions of universal shortage of ICU beds[12,13,28,29] and in conditions of expensive cost of ICU care worldwide.[30]

Triage decision requires cautious clinical judgment to balance the clinical benefit of ICU care with associated risks and costs. Even if ICUs are often the only place where HF patients in critical condition can receive life-saving therapies, ICU care settings are associated with a high risk of iatrogenic complications, such as venous thromboembolism, upper gastrointestinal bleeding, and hospital-acquired infection with multidrug-resistant pathogens.[31–33] These complications contribute to reduced quality of life of HF patients, beyond that attributed to HF solely.[34] Additionally, HF patients who require ICU care are often discharged with a low rate or suboptimal regimen of oral HF therapies.[35]

Recently, a consensus study[20] by the Heart Failure Association of the European Society of Cardiology and the European Society of Emergency Medicine offered objective criteria for ICU admission in high-risk AHF patients, and these include: RR greater than 25 breaths/min, Sao_2 less than 90%, use of accessory muscles for breathing, need for intubation, SBP less than

90 mm Hg, and signs of hypoperfusion. These criteria are based, however, on expert opinion consensus and were not prospectively validated.

Future research is needed to estimate the clinical probability of ICU admission based on clinical variables collected at presentation. Risk scores can help identify a high-risk AHF population that could potentially be directed to an ICU environment. In the Acute Decompensated Heart Failure National Registry (ADHERE),[36] a subgroup of patients with concomitant SBP less than 115 mm Hg, serum urea nitrogen greater than 43 mg/dL, and creatinine greater than 2.75 mg/dL had an in-hospital mortality of 22%, suggesting potential benefit for direct ICU admission. In the RO-AHFS registry, some of the variables commonly collected at admission, including, age, low SBP, low left ventricular ejection fraction, and low serum sodium, predict the necessity for ICU admission in patients hospitalized for AHF, but none of these variables was associated with in-hospital ACM in ICU setting, suggesting that the clinical characteristics at the time point of ICU admission may differ compared with those collected at initial presentation because clinical stability of AHFS patients may improve or worsen as result of in-hospital therapies.

CLINICAL RESEARCH IN THE INTENSIVE CARE UNIT SETTING

As a common area for the disposition of the critically ill patients with HF, the ICU also provides access to a large number of patients with a high expected event rate and would, therefore, be an excellent environment from which to conduct critical care research. Potential areas of research include noninvasive methods of hemodynamic monitoring, identifying risk factors for the development of left ventricular dysfunction in the setting of sepsis, determinants of RV dysfunction, and assessing the impact of noncardiac comorbidities on outcomes.

The lack of guideline recommendations supporting individual interventions that would require an ICU as well as wide European differences in facilities, however, may contribute to considerable variation in clinical practice. Consequently, before conducting more elaborate research in ICU environments, national specific characteristics should be identified, including number of ICU and CCU beds of the total bed capacity of the hospital, ICU/CCU staffing, and a more detailed description of the available procedural interventions in the ICU/CCU. More research is needed to understand how the differing numbers of ICU/CCU beds have an impact on practice protocols and finally on patient outcomes. Because a decision to transfer patients to an ICU is multifactorial, additional research is needed to clarify the reason and type of ICU transfer as well as European practices in terms of medical staffing.

EUROPEAN PERSPECTIVES ON TRAINING AND EDUCATION IN CRITICAL CARE

The requirement to manage critically ill patients in different care settings and changing demographic and clinical characteristics of patients admitted to critical care areas[37] have resulted in recognition of the need for supplementary training for physicians taking care of these patients. Furthermore, to optimize the delivery of patient-centered care to critically ill patients, potentially in high-stress and

---

Box 1
Competencies needed for certification in acute cardiac care subspecialty

- Diagnosis, assessment, and management of cardiovascular emergencies
- Diagnosis, assessment, and management of critically ill patient
- Prevention and management of multiorgan dysfunction in the critically ill cardiac patient
- To know strengths and limitations of investigations and interventions performed in ICU/CCU
- Competency with operation of available equipment
- Competency in the management of infections, sedation, and analgesia
- To evaluate the risk of patient transportation
- Determination and planning of more long term management as part of a step-down strategy from ICU/ICCU
- To participate at end-of-life decision making process

Data from European Society of Cardiology. The ESC Core Curriculum for Acute Cardiac Care (2014). Available at: http://www.escardio.org/communities/Working-Groups/acute-cardiac-care/Documents/ESC-Curriculum-Training-Intensive-ACCEurope.pdf. Accessed June 29, 2015.

time-pressured environments, multidisciplinary teamwork is crucial in ICU and CCU departments.[38]

Recognizing the developments in both intensive care medicine and acute cardiology that have occurred over recent years and the requirement for a multisystem approach to critically ill patients, the European Society of Cardiology and the Acute Cardiac Care Working Group elaborated on an acute cardiac care curriculum with the intention to create a new subspecialty for cardiologists.[39] A total of at least 21 months of intensive care training is needed for certification in the acute cardiac care subspecialty. Completion of the curriculum should offer trained cardiologists knowledge, skills, behavior, and attitudes for acting independently in the critical care environment (**Box 1**).

SUMMARY

Data from contemporary HF registries suggest that ICU admission rates differ considerably across the Europe. Wide variations across Europe regarding local protocols and facilities available in ICUs and CCUs may contribute to these regional differences. Despite large variations in treatment practices, the subset of European patients managed in the ICUs had similar high rates of ACM.

Triaging AHF patients to the appropriate level of care at presentation may potentially result in improvements in quality of care and in-hospital outcomes, but future research is required to prospectively validate ICU triage algorithms.

In addition, application of high-quality strategies to these high-risk cardiac patients requires medical personnel with adequate competencies in acute cardiac care and an ongoing collaboration between cardiology and intensive care medicine.

REFERENCES

1. McMurray JJ, Adamopoulos S, Anker SD, et al. ESC guidelines for the diagnosis and treatment of acute and chronic heart failure 2012: The Task Force for the Diagnosis and Treatment of Acute and Chronic Heart Failure 2012 of the European Society of Cardiology. Developed in collaboration with the Heart Failure Association (HFA) of the ESC. Eur J Heart Fail 2012;14(8):803–69.

2. Gheorghiade M, Zannad F, Sopko G, et al, for the International Working Group on Acute Heart Failure Syndromes. Acute heart failure syndromes: current state and framework for future research. Circulation 2005;112:3958–68.

3. Hasin Y, Danchin N, Filippatos G, et al. Recommendations for the structure, organization, and operation of intensive cardiac care units. Eur Heart J 2005;26: 1676–82.

4. Wunsch H, Angus DC, Harrison DA, et al. Variation in critical care services across North America and Western Europe. Crit Care Med 2008;36:2787–93. e1–9.

5. Gray A, Goodacre S, Newby DE, et al. Noninvasive ventilation in acute cardiogenic pulmonary edema. N Engl J Med 2008;359:142–51.

6. Deepa C, Muralidhar K. Renal replacement therapy in ICU. J Anaesthesiol Clin Pharmacol 2012;28(3): 386–96.

7. Pronovost PJ, Angus DC, Dorman T, et al. Physician staffing patterns and clinical outcomes in critically ill patients. A systematic review. JAMA 2002;288: 2151–62.

8. O'Malley RG, Olenchock B, Bohula-May E, et al. Organization and staffing practices in US cardiac intensive care units: a survey on behalf of the American Heart Association Writing Group on the Evolution of Critical Care Cardiology. Eur Heart J Acute Cardiovasc Care 2013;2:3.

9. Chioncel O, Ambrosy AP, Filipescu D, et al. Patterns of intensive care unit admissions in patients hospitalized for heart failure: insights from the RO-AHFS registry. J Cardiovasc Med (Hagerstown) 2015;16(5): 331–40.

10. Zannad F, Mebazaa A, Juilliere Y, et al. Clinical profile, contemporary management and one-year mortality in patients with severe acute heart failure syndromes: the EFICA study. Eur J Heart Fail 2006;8:697–705.

11. Follath F, Yilmaz MB, Delgado JF, et al. Clinical presentation, management and outcomes in the Acute Heart Failure Global Survey of Standard Treatment (ALARM-HF). Intensive Care Med 2011;37(4):619–26.

12. Rhodes A, Ferdinande P, Flaatten H, et al. The variability of critical care bed numbers in Europe. Intensive Care Med 2012;38:1647–53.

13. Adhikari NK, Fowler RA, Bhagwanjee S, et al. Critical care and the global burden of critical illness in adults. Lancet 2010;376:1339–46.

14. van Diepen S, Podder M, Hernandez AF, et al. Acute decompensated heart failure patients admitted to critical care units: Insights from ASCEND-HF. Int J Cardiol 2014;177:840–6.

15. Siirila-Waris K, Lassus J, Melin J, et al. Characteristics, outcomes, and predictors of 1-year mortality in patients hospitalized for acute heart failure. Eur Heart J 2006;27:3011–7.

16. Nieminen MS, Brutsaert D, Dickstein K, et al. EuroHeart Failure Survey II (EHFS II): a survey on hospitalized acute heart failure patients: description of population. Eur Heart J 2006;27: 2725–36.

17. Logeart D, Isnard R, Resche-Rigon M, et al, on behalf of the working group on Heart Failure of the

French Society of Cardiology. Current aspects of the spectrum of acute heart failure syndromes in a real-life setting: the OFICA study. Eur J Heart Fail 2013; 15:363–478.

18. Oliva F, Mortara A, Cacciatore G, et al, on the behalf of the IN-HF Outcome Investigators. Acute heart failure patient profiles, management and in-hospital outcome: results of the Italian Registry on Heart Failure Outcome. Eur J Heart Fail 2012;14:1208–17.

19. Chioncel O, Vinereanu D, Datcu M, et al. The Romanian Acute Heart Failure Syndromes (RO-AHFS) registry. Am Heart J 2011;162:142–53.e1.

20. Mebazaa A, Yilmaz MB, Levy P, et al. Recommendations on pre-hospital & hospital management of acute heart failure: a consensus paper from the Heart Failure Association of the European Society of Cardiology, the European Society of Emergency Medicine and the Society of Academic Emergency Medicine. Eur J Heart Fail 2015. http://dx.doi.org/10.1002/ejhf.289.

21. Ambrosy A, Gheorghiade M, Bubenek S, et al. The predictive value of transaminases at admission in patients hospitalized for heart failure: findings from the RO-AHFS registry. Eur Heart J Acute Cardiovasc Care 2013;2(2):99–108.

22. Kazory A. Hyponatremia in heart failure: revisiting pathophysiology and therapeutic strategies. Clin Cardiol 2010;33:322–9.

23. Abid O, Akca S, Haji-Michael P, et al. Strong vasopressor support may be futile in the intensive care unit patient with multiple organ failure. Crit Care Med 2000;28(4):947–9.

24. Cox CE, Martinu T, Sathy SJ, et al. Expectations and outcomes of prolonged mechanical ventilation. Crit Care Med 2009;37(11):2888.

25. Hayashi Y, Morisawa K, Klompas M, et al. Toward improved surveillance: the impact of ventilator-associated complications on length of stay and antibiotic use in patients in intensive care units. Clin Infect Dis 2013;56:471–7.

26. Chalfin DB, Trzeciak S, Likourezos A, et al. Impact of delayed transfer of critically ill patients from the emergency department to the intensive care unit. Crit Care Med 2007;35:1477–83.

27. Zimmerman JE, Kramer AA. A model for identifying patients who may not need intensive care unit admission. J Crit Care 2010;25:205–13.

28. Sinuff T, Kahnamoui K, Cook DJ, et al, Values Ethics and Rationing in Critical Care Task Force. Rationing critical care beds: a systematic review. Crit Care Med 2004;32(7):1588–97.

29. Stelfox HT, Hemmelgarn BR, Bagshaw SM, et al. Intensive care unit bed availability and outcomes for hospitalized patients with sudden clinical deterioration. Arch Intern Med 2012;172(6):467–74.

30. Milbrandt EB, Kersten A, Rahim MT, et al. Growth of intensive care unit resource use and its estimated cost in Medicare. Crit Care Med 2008;36:2504–10.

31. Smith WR, Poses RM, Donna K, et al. Prognostic judgments and triage decisions for patients with acute congestive heart failure. Chest 2002;121: 1610–7.

32. Giraud T, Dhainaut JF, Vaxelaire JF, et al. Iatrogenic complications in adult intensive care units: a prospective two center study. Crit Care Med 1993;21: 40–51.

33. Saint S, Matthay MA. Risk reduction in the intensive care unit. Am J Med 1998;105:515–23.

34. Oeyen SG, Vandijck DM, Benoit DD, et al. Quality of life after intensive care: a systematic review of the literature. Crit Care Med 2010;38:2386–400.

35. Bell CM, Brener SS, Gunraj N, et al. Association of ICU or hospital admission with unintentional discontinuation of medications for chronic diseases. JAMA 2011;306:840–7.

36. Fonarow GC, Adams KF Jr, Abraham WT, et al, Adhere Scientific Advisory Committee Study Group, Investigators. Risk stratification for in-hospital mortality in acutely decompensated heart failure: classification and regression tree analysis. JAMA 2005; 293(5):572–80.

37. Katz JN, Turer AT, Bicker RC. Cardiology and the critical care crisis. A Perspective. J Am Coll Cardiol 2007;49:1279–82.

38. Gillebert TC, Brooks N, Fontes-Carvalho R, et al, on behalf of Task Force Members Committee for Education. ESC core curriculum for the general cardiologist (2013). Eur Heart J 2013;34:2381–411.

39. European Society of Cardiology. The ESC Core Curriculum for Acute Cardiac Care (2014). Available at: http://www.escardio.org/static_file/Escardio/Subspecialty/ACCA/core-curriculum-ACCA-2014-FINAL.pdf. Accessed July 29, 2015.

United States Postal Service

Statement of Ownership, Management, and Circulation
(All Periodicals Publications Except Requester Publications)

1. Publication Title: Heart Failure Clinics

2. Publication Number: 0 2 5 5 - 0 5 5

3. Filing Date: 9/18/15

4. Issue Frequency: Jan, Apr, Jul, Oct

5. Number of Issues Published Annually: 4

6. Annual Subscription Price: $235.00

7. Complete Mailing Address of Known Office of Publication (Not printer) (Street, city, county, state, and ZIP+4®)

Elsevier Inc.
360 Park Avenue South
New York, NY 10010-1710

Contact Person: Stephen R. Bushing

Telephone (Include area code): 215-239-3688

8. Complete Mailing Address of Headquarters or General Business Office of Publisher (Not printer)

Elsevier Inc., 360 Park Avenue South, New York, NY 10010-1710

9. Full Names and Complete Mailing Addresses of Publisher, Editor, and Managing Editor (Do not leave blank)

Publisher (Name and complete mailing address)

Linda Belfus, Elsevier Inc., 1600 John F. Kennedy Blvd., Suite 1800, Philadelphia, PA 19103

Editor (Name and complete mailing address)

Adrianne Brigido, Elsevier Inc., 1600 John F. Kennedy Blvd., Suite 1800, Philadelphia, PA 19103-2899

Managing Editor (Name and complete mailing address)

Lauren Boyle, Elsevier Inc., 1600 John F. Kennedy Blvd., Suite 1800, Philadelphia, PA 19103-2899

10. Owner (Do not leave blank. If the publication is owned by a corporation, give the name and address of the corporation immediately followed by the names and addresses of all stockholders owning or holding 1 percent or more of the total amount of stock. If not owned by a corporation, give the names and addresses of the individual owners. If owned by a partnership or other unincorporated firm, give its name and address as well as those of each individual owner. If the publication is published by a nonprofit organization, give its name and address.)

Full Name	Complete Mailing Address
Wholly owned subsidiary of	1600 John F. Kennedy Blvd., Ste. 1800
Reed/Elsevier, US holdings	Philadelphia, PA 19103-2899

11. Known Bondholders, Mortgagees, and Other Security Holders Owning or Holding 1 Percent or More of Total Amount of Bonds, Mortgages, or Other Securities. If none, check box ☐ None

Full Name	Complete Mailing Address
N/A	

12. Tax Status (For completion by nonprofit organizations authorized to mail at nonprofit rates) (Check one)
The purpose, function, and nonprofit status of this organization and the exempt status for federal income tax purposes:
☐ Has Not Changed During Preceding 12 Months
☐ Has Changed During Preceding 12 Months (Publisher must submit explanation of change with this statement)

13. Publication Title: Heart Failure Clinics

14. Issue Date for Circulation Data Below: July 2015

15. Extent and Nature of Circulation			Average No. Copies Each Issue During Preceding 12 Months	No. Copies of Single Issue Published Nearest to Filing Date
a. Total Number of Copies (Net press run)			191	170
b. Legitimate Paid and/Or Requested Distribution (By Mail and Outside the Mail)	(1)	Mailed Outside-County Paid/Requested Mail Subscriptions stated on PS Form 3541. (Include paid distribution above nominal rate, advertiser's proof copies and exchange copies)	37	37
	(2)	Mailed In-County Paid/Requested Mail Subscriptions stated on PS Form 3541. (Include paid distribution above nominal rate, advertiser's proof copies and exchange copies)		
	(3)	Paid Distribution Outside the Mails Including Sales Through Dealers And Carriers, Street Vendors, Counter Sales, and Other Paid Distribution Outside USPS®	17	19
	(4)	Paid Distribution by Other Classes of Mail Through the USPS (e.g. First-Class Mail®)		
c. Total Paid and or Requested Circulation (Sum of 15b (1), (2), (3), and (4))			54	56
d. Free or Nominal Rate Distribution (By Mail and Outside the Mail)	(1)	Free or Nominal Rate Outside-County Copies included on PS Form 3541	66	64
	(2)	Free or Nominal Rate In-County Copies included on PS Form 3541		
	(3)	Free or Nominal Rate Copies mailed at Other classes Through the USPS (e.g. First-Class Mail®)		
	(4)	Free or Nominal Rate Distribution Outside the Mail (Carriers or Other means)		
e. Total Nonrequested Distribution (Sum of 15d (1), (2), (3) and (4))			66	64
f. Total Distribution (Sum of 15c and 15e)			120	120
g. Copies not Distributed (See instructions to publishers #4 (page #3))			71	50
h. Total (Sum of 15f and g)			191	170
i. Percent Paid and/or Requested Circulation (15c divided by 15f times 100)			45.00%	46.67%

* If you are claiming electronic copies go to line 16 on page 3. If you are not claiming Electronic copies, skip to line 17 on page 3.

16. Electronic Copy Circulation	Average No. Copies Each Issue During Preceding 12 Months	No. Copies of Single Issue Published Nearest to Filing Date
a. Paid Electronic Copies		
b. Total paid Print Copies (Line 15c) + Paid Electronic copies (Line 16a)		
c. Total Print Distribution (Line 15f) + Paid Electronic Copies (Line 16a)		
d. Percent Paid (Both Print & Electronic copies) (16b divided by 16c X 100)		

☐ I certify that 50% of all my distributed copies (electronic and print) are paid above a nominal price

17. Publication of Statement of Ownership
If the publication is a general publication, publication of this statement is required. Will be printed in the _October 2015_ issue of this publication.

18. Signature and Title of Editor, Publisher, Business Manager, or Owner

Stephen R. Bushing – Inventory Distribution Coordinator

I certify that all information furnished on this form is true and complete. I understand that anyone who furnishes false or misleading information on this form or who omits material or information requested on the form may be subject to criminal sanctions (including fines and imprisonment) and/or civil sanctions (including civil penalties).

Date: September 18, 2015

PS Form 3526, July 2014 (Page 1 of 3) (Instructions Page 3)) PSN 7530-01-000-9931 PRIVACY NOTICE: See our Privacy policy in www.usps.com

PS Form 3526, July 2014 (Page 3 of 3)